Praise for *Left / Write // Hook*

By no choice of their own, survivors of childhood sexual abuse spend the entirety of their lives 'in the ring', fighting. *Left / Write // Hook* offers visceral insight into survivors' fierce, compelling and ultimately triumphant stories.

Dr Joy Townsend, Learning Consent

Donna Lyon has the ability to get women to open up and reveal all, and in the process begin the journey to healing. Boxing is a violent sport, but projects like *Left / Write // Hook* take the violence out of it, so that it becomes therapeutic and gives you power.

**Tommy Hopkins, Fitlife Boxing Club,
Melbourne Australia**

In 25+ years of working with people who have experienced childhood sexual abuse, I have come to understand the need to assist people *to physically move through, as well as speak about*, the trauma in order to lessen the hold that the impacts that the abuse can have on one's life — *Left / Write // Hook* does both with powerful effectiveness.

Maria Vucko, (BA BSW MSW AMHSW)

LEFT / WRITE // HOOK

Survivor Stories from a Creative Arts Boxing and Writing Project

Edited by **Donna Lyon** and **Claire Gaskin**

Loving Healing Press
Ann Arbor, Michigan

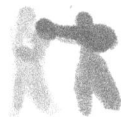

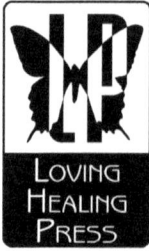

Left / Write // Hook: Survivor Stories
from a Creative Arts Boxing and Writing Project

Published by: Loving Healing Press
                 5145 Pontiac Trail
                 Ann Arbor, MI 48105
                 www.LHPress.com
                 info@LHPress.com

Library of Congress Cataloging-in-Publication Data
Names: Lyon, Donna, 1980 — editor.
Title: Left/Write//Hook: Survivor Stories from
                 a Creative Arts Boxing and Writing Project
                 [edited by] Donna Lyon.
Other titles: Left Write Hook
Identifiers: LCCN 2021026340 (print)
                 LCCN 2021026341 (ebook)

ISBN 978-1-61599-580-6 paperback
ISBN 978-1-61599-581-3 hardcover
ISBN 978-1-61599-582-0 eBook

Subjects: LCSH: Adult child sexual abuse victims.
                 Creative writing — Therapeutic use.
                 Boxing — Therapeutic use
Classification: LCC RC569.5.A28 L44 2021 (print)
                 LCC RC569.5.A28 (ebook)
                 DDC 362.76/4--dc23

LC record available at: lccn.loc.gov/2021026340
LC ebook record available at: lccn.loc.gov/202102634

Cover design by Nuttshell Graphics

Use of Sting Logo approved by Sting International Pty Ltd

Punch Boxing Gloves used with the permission of Punch Equipment

Individual stories copyright retained by the authors,
who assert their rights to be known as the authors of the work.

'Common Terms Used in the Book' is used with the express permission
of Sidran Traumatic Stress Institute (c) 2021
www.sidran.org/glossary/ and **www.sidran.org/wp-content/
uploads/2018/11/What-is-a-dissociative-disorder.pdf**

Acknowledgements

**This book was made possible through
the funding and support of the:**

Creativity and Wellbeing Hallmark Research Initiative
and Research Development Grant of University
of Melbourne, Faculty of Fine Arts and Music

Thank you's

**Thank you to the following contributors
and supporters of this project:**

Mischa's Boxing Central and Mischa Merz

University of Melbourne research team:
Shannon Owen, Ella Sowinska, Dr. Margaret Osborne,
Dr. Khandis Blake, Bruna Andrades, Dr Steve Thomas

University of Melbourne Faculty of Fine Arts
and Music VCA Film and Television

Tommy Hopkins and Fitlife Boxing Gym

Amir Attalla

Shannon Anderson

Acknowledgment of Country

We acknowledge the people of the Kulin nation, the traditional custodians of the lands that this book was developed and produced on. We pay our respects to their Elders past, present and future. We recognise that sovereignty has never been ceded.

As we share our experiences of trauma, we recognise the traumatic histories of dispossession and colonisation of Australia's First Peoples. We believe it is untenable to talk about issues of abuse and trauma in Australia without acknowledging these histories and their ongoing impacts.

Trigger Warning

This book is written by adult survivors of childhood sexual abuse who are openly declaring the effects, feelings, ramifications and manifestations of their abuse. Our writing is honest, brutal and raw and at times we use profanity. Nothing was censored in these workshops and so you might find what we share is triggering. If you do, we encourage you to take a break, practice self-care or seek the relevant support that you might need.

Sexual abuse is disgusting. Talking about it can cause discomfort from others and often from within ourselves. If you are a survivor and have not yet shared your story, we hope that our writings and thoughts might resonate with you and provide you with some hope and comfort that you are not alone.

Contents

Introduction 13

The Project 16

Group positioning statement 17

A note about our writings 18

A note about our temporal (temporary) self 19

Common terms used in this book 20

**The experience of *Left/Write//Hook* (LWH)
from the workshop participants** 23

Before 23

During 27

After 33

ROUND 1 37

About Round 1 38

Round 1 Writing Prompts 39

I am here because | Being here 40

I connected and… | To punch is to…
Hand to cheek, I step, I punch, I… 47

There is no wonder | If it hadn't happened | Now that 54

The virus | My mother is a foot 69

Isolation | Madness 74

Vulnerability | Disgust | Shame 79

Mind | Body 92

I Remember | Being Believed Means 103

Recovery | Healing | Things I Like 108

Power | Fighting Back | Compassion 117

The last eight weeks 120

ROUND 2

ROUND 2   131

About Round 2   132

Round 2 Writing Prompts   133

I am back here because | I begin again | Today   134

Being a Survivor | Denial   143

Trusting the process | Being on Guard | Relaxation   147

When I listen | I listened | Two feet on the ground
Being present   154

Write a conversation between you and your nervous system
Write a love letter to a part of your body
Write all the things you hate and all the things you love   165

Reclaiming me | Self-esteem   170

He / She / They / I pushed... | I turned...   175

I thought I was going to
It's hard to speak out because | What it takes   181

Intimacy | Effects of my abuse
Write a letter to your inner child | What is meaningful?   186

Trauma   196

Silence   198

Writing + Boxing =   201

ROUND 3   205

About Round 3   206

Round 3 Writing Prompts   207

I return | This time | I feel | Developing a practice   208

My commitment to self is
Trusting myself | Trusting others   215

I was told | Ways I was trained to be powerless
Ways I have reclaimed myself | Feeling powerful   220

Things I've felt responsible for
My reality | The way I see things   235

I see you | When you see me | I hear you   244

Rage | I am angry   250

Being there for others | In its place | On the way   254

I pretend | I was tricked | Don't disturb   263

Preferred ways of being | Prescribed ways of being   273

The Unknown | The Atmosphere   277

I say goodbye to | The last eight weeks   281

What has the group given to you that you
would like other survivors to know about?   287

Epilogue   291

Contributor Bios   294

Introduction

The first time I got punched in the face in a training session, I cried afterwards in my car.

It wasn't so much that it hurt, it was the shock. I froze, but I was encouraged to punch back. Boxing brought up buried emotion deep inside of me. As much as it didn't seem very tough to shed tears, the process felt part of my healing journey.

I started boxing in my mid-thirties. I was angry and I knew it was directly related to my childhood sexual abuse and trauma. Secretly I felt drawn to boxing, its visceral nature. The prospect of hitting someone in the face and maybe even knocking them out excited me. Little did I know that within a few months of signing up to a boxing gym, I would be training for my first fight. I went on an 18-month beginners' journey into the world of master's boxing, an amateur division for those aged 35 and older.

My first fight was my most memorable. I fought a woman in her fifties who had a gold tooth. She was tough with a mean look in her eye and I loved every bit of the experience. The brilliance of naivete! It was a split decision, but the final point went to her. I lost, but I didn't care. I felt elated. The feeling was short lived, as I fought another three times and lost.

The more I took fighting into the competitive space, the more disempowered I became. Lack of experience was a key factor, but performance anxiety overtook me. I practiced mindfulness (a difficult task for someone who had experienced dissociation her whole life). I tried to visualise winning and work with my inner children to quell the fear and voices, but to no avail. I dissociated in the ring. As I lost fights, louder came the chant of negative voices within me. The unconscious beliefs I had about being a failure, a loser and worthless started to overtake me. I kept powering on, fighting hard to battle through the negativity. Fighting became a metaphor for recovering from my abuse.

The training motivated me; I trained five times a week. I started running to increase my cardio. I got a trainer and we spoke daily about my routine and mental health. I remember driving to a sparring session with him one day. He said, "You are the most difficult person I have ever trained." I looked confused. He went on; "Most people when they get hit, punch straight back. When you get hit, you just freeze." I responded that it was instinctual. I would dissociate. Boxing triggered the feeling of the loss of control and anxiety associated with my past trauma. But I kept returning to it, determined to crack the code to release me from the bind and break through to the other side. Yet my trauma continued to undermine my boxing. I struggled to think logically and stay calm, let alone be present. I loved how boxing challenged me to try and overcome these fears, but the self-criticism, judgement, disappointment, and confusion connected to trying to win became harder to reconcile. After my final loss, I ended up having a win, in a small interclub fight. The stakes weren't as high as the other fights and I didn't even know it was a win/ lose fight. I took home a medal and it felt bittersweet. At least I could say I won one, I guess.

I loved being a fighter, even if I wasn't very good at it. I have mostly been determined to fight my way through life and work through things, rather than running from them. After a period of reflection, I knew that what I enjoyed about boxing hadn't changed. Hitting a bag hard, training, sweating, focusing on my body and breath, movement, and speed; toying with being relaxed and calm, yet sharp and on point. Boxing is a delicate interplay between the physical and the mental. It is both art and skill. It is these elements that have kept me coming back to this sport.

Although my fighting career was over, I began to wonder if there were other women like me; survivors, who could use boxing as a recovery tool, a mode of empowerment to express their trauma. I wanted to not only box with survivors, I wanted to hear their stories and share my experiences of trauma. My background is as an educator, a filmmaker, and an arts practitioner, so the juxtaposition of writing and boxing, although contradictory, felt right to me. I wanted to know what would happen if you put a bunch of survivors in a gym to firstly write about their trauma and then learn the basics of boxing to channel the feelings. And so, in 2018, I set up *Left/Write//Hook* and ran the project independently. In 2019, I became a level one boxing coach and in 2020, I took the project into the research space at University of Melbourne, where I lecture in Producing for Film and Television.

Left/Write//Hook is not about becoming a writer, or a fighter. I believe survivors need to give their trauma expression. I believe survivors are already fighters. I knew what it was like to fight through shame, negative thinking, addiction, toxic beliefs and even for the will to want to survive and live life. I knew that other survivors felt the same. Journal writing had helped me in the past, but I found it hard to do. I felt sleepy after I wrote, as though expressing the trauma and then just leaving it there on paper was only one part of the process. I needed to give the words emotion, the memories a purpose. I needed to move the trauma through my mind, then into and out of my body.

I set up *Left/Write//Hook* for me and I was grateful when others joined. I am even more thankful to be growing this project in tandem with others, particularly the survivors whose work is featured in this book, all of whom have boldly stepped into the ring to share their trauma. This project has a life of its own. It has given me a purpose and I feel supported and accountable. My heart breaks when I hear each person share their writings. I connect to the heartache of my dissociated and repressed trauma through the words of those in the group. I develop compassion and empathy for my selves and others. The pain I have been carrying all these years is shared and it suddenly develops perspective and is given new context. I can reveal all of me and the fragments of my identity, yet I am gently encouraged to stay strong and keep going. It's an understanding that life is not easy, but a reminder that joy is still to be found.

Donna Lyon

The Project

Left/Write//Hook is an evidence-based project that aims to support and amplify the voice and agency of female and gender diverse survivors of childhood sexual abuse and trauma through writing and boxing. It is founded and led by boxer, academic, researcher, producer and survivor of extreme sexual and mental abuse, Donna Lyon.

This book is a co-curation of writings from the participants who came together in 2020 to form part of a creative arts research project into the *Left/Write//Hook* program. The project was funded through a grant from University of Melbourne Creativity and Wellbeing Research Institute, situated within the Faculty of Fine Arts and Music. This iteration of *Left/Write//Hook* brought together an interdisciplinary research team and mixed methods research design to explore the impact of the program on the participant's wellbeing and sense of agency. This included a documentary filmmaker who, with a small team, filmed the program, with the intent of producing a long form documentary film. Allowing a camera into the space to document the process was very confronting for most of the people in the room. It meant essentially 'coming out' as a survivor and claiming this label in a public manner.

At the end of week two of Round One, Covid-19 hit. The group were situated in Melbourne, Australia and quickly went into lockdown. Ranked as one of the longest and toughest lockdowns in the world, the group were to spend approximately seven months in domestic and online environments. After consulting with the research team, in week three, the project moved online to zoom. The research component ran officially for eight weeks, however Lyon continued to run *Left/Write//Hook* over three rounds with the participants, throughout 2020.

As of the time of writing, the filmmaking research team and survivors are continuing to work on the documentary and capture aspects of our journey, including the many book meetings we have had to formulate this selection of our writings. A journal article has been released to report the research findings and the *Left/Write//Hook* program continues to develop and take shape to reach more survivors.

Group positioning statement

We are a group of people with lived experience of childhood sexual abuse, this is the context in which we came together. Our experiences are different, but the effects of our abuse have been resoundingly similar.

We offer insight into what it means to live as a survivor. The adverse effects of childhood sexual abuse are long term. Trauma lives in the body, and it needs to be expressed.

We are a group of white, female and gender diverse survivors, whose ages range from 28 to 55. Our abuse ranges from incest, attacks from people in our social circles, to assaults by complete strangers, through to organisational, institutional, and ritual abuse. We do not speak for or represent all survivors.

We came together in 2020 as part of a creative arts research project combining boxing and writing. Our trauma responses include depression, anxiety, low self-esteem, suicidal ideation, eating disorders, body dysmorphia, addiction, suicide attempts and difficulties forming and maintaining interpersonal relationships.

Some of us have been institutionalised, some have not. Many of us have experienced stigma, and financial hardship. Some of us even have PhDs. Many of us are professionals, others cannot work due to the struggles of dealing with the daily effects of our abuse. Some of us have children. Others are in heterosexual or same-sex relationships, or have difficulty being in a relationship. Some of us are still in close contact with our families, others have had to sever all ties.

Some of us have faith in God. Some of us have a personal spirituality. Some of us find the concept of God difficult to embrace. Others have completely rejected organised religion due to the part it has played in our lifelong trauma.

We have co-curated and created this book together. We have taken responsibility for what writings we were comfortable sharing and how we wanted to be named and identified.

We acknowledge that there are many parts to each of us, within the group and as a whole.

Any allegations made against any individual in this book have not been admitted to by the alleged wrongdoer/s.

A note about our writings

The writings in this book were written as a free form response to a writing prompt. No structural format was assigned. This style may be referred to as prose poetry, allowing for the combination of the poetic and prose form to reveal itself through creative writing. Each writer was encouraged to express themselves in whatever way they liked, and each writing was considered a form of artistic expression. All writing was seen as being instinctively *right*. At times the writing is from deep within the writer's subconscious and does not follow the bounds of language and expression. Punctuation may not exist, tense may change, and words may be spontaneous, creative, and broad. The process of writing may sometimes contain a pattern, other times, it is purely about bypassing the censoring parts of our minds.

A note about our temporal (temporary) self

Every workshop began with a check-in. We sat together and were asked one at a time how we were going. This is simple and like a lot of simple things it is very profound. It is an invitation to check-in not check-out and take on a role or abandon self to be there for others. I was listened to; the others were there for me and I listened to them. It was like checking into a hotel, but this hotel was not a holiday it was an opportunity to reside in my authentic self, not a self in recovery not a self that had to play a role as a professional or friend or mother, lover, daughter, sister, but an authentic self, there to tell the truth of my experiences. This was a place I could be honest and not be shut down or silenced. I would not be judged, doubted, interrogated, discredited, dismissed, and disbelieved. Here was a place I could talk about what I could not talk about in any other setting. Some people can talk about their life openly without fear of causing other people vicarious trauma, I cannot.

In this context of trust, we were given writing prompts. I wrote without editing myself, I wrote freely. I wrote about how I felt at the time. I do not need to identify with what I wrote as definitive; I do not have to identify with it at all. My writings represent what I was thinking and feeling at specific moments in time, not what I think and feel at all times. My writing does not represent all that I am, it is writing, it is thinking and feeling, it is not me. It represents a temporary self at best. Once it is written I have already changed. I am never finished, complete or containable. I am forever in becoming, I am irreducible.

Claire Gaskin

Common terms used in this book[1]

Dissociation

The separation of ideas, feelings, information, identity, or memories that would normally go together. Dissociation exists on a continuum: At one end are mild dissociative experiences common to most people (such as daydreaming or highway hypnosis) and at the other extreme is severe chronic dissociation, such as Dissociative Identity Disorder (formerly known as Multiple Personality Disorder) and other dissociative disorders. Dissociation appears to be a normal process used to handle trauma that over time becomes reinforced and develops into maladaptive coping.

Dissociative Identity Disorder (DID)

Tragically, ongoing traumatic conditions such as abuse, community violence, war, or painful medical procedures are not one-time events. For people repeatedly exposed to these experiences, especially in childhood, dissociation is an extremely effective coping "skill." However, it can become a double-edged sword. It can protect them from awareness of the pain in the short-run, but a person who dissociates often may find in the long-run his or her sense of personal history and identity is affected. For some people, dissociation is so frequent it results in serious pathology, relationship difficulties, and inability to function, especially when under stress.

Fragment *(often expressed by the writers as selves or parts or inner child or children)*

Within the personality system of a person who has a dissociative disorder, a fragment is a dissociated part of that person which has limited function and is less distinct or developed than a personality state. Usually, a fragment has a consistent emotional and behavioral response to specific situations. For example, a fragment may handle the expression of feelings through drawing.

Ritual abuse

While not necessarily satanic, ritual abuse generally involves cult-like or religious rituals and mind control in addition to sexual, physical and/or psychological abuse. "...repeated abuse over an extended period of time. The physical abuse is severe, sometimes including torture and killing. The sexual abuse is usually painful, humiliating, intended as a means of gaining dominance over the victim. The psychological abuse is devastating and involves the use of ritual indoctrination. It includes mind control techniques which convey to the victim a profound terror of the cult members...most victims are in a state of terror, mind control and dissociation." Report of the Ritual Abuse Task Force, Los Angeles County Commission for Women, 1991, p. 1.

System

A descriptive term for all the aspects or parts of the mind in an individual with DID (MPD). This includes personality states, memories, feelings, ego states, entities, and any other way of describing dissociated aspects of an individual. Understanding the parts as a system rather than as separate personality states provides an important frame of reference for treatment. Also called internal system or personality system.

[1]Used with the express permission of Sidran Traumatic Stress Institute (C) 2021
www.sidran.org/glossary/ and
www.sidran.org/wp-content/uploads/2018/11/What-is-a-dissociative-disorder.pdf

The experience of *Left / Write // Hook* (LWH) from the workshop participants

Before

Claire speaks...

Before the workshops I felt isolated

After the workshops I feel a sense of community and conviction

Before the workshops I felt enormous fear of memories

After the workshops I feel memories are breakthroughs into coherence

Before the workshops I felt shame I felt sick of having
    the worst story in any given room

After the workshops I feel less shame and more solidarity

Before the workshops I felt stuck in pretending to be alright

After the workshops I feel more ground underneath me

Before the workshops I felt on the verge of realisation

After the workshops I feel more certain of the life I have made

Before the workshops I felt remaining hidden
    was the most important occupation

After the workshops I feel I can look without looking away

Before the workshops I felt flinchy and reactive in public

After the workshops I feel I can occupy the space I take up and be still

Julie speaks...

Before I started at LWH my life was turbulent. My mental health was all over the place. I didn't see myself as a survivor or a victim, just somebody who endured horrific child sexual abuse at the hands of some horrible men and boys. I thought it was normal and that it happened to most people. How very wrong I was!

I was staying at a place called PARC (Prevention and Recovery Care) and my partner called me and told me about Donna's article in the paper. I really didn't think it was for me, but I thought about it and said FUCK IT I will give it a try. I am very overweight and very unfit and of course was very scared. That was two years ago. Before my first session I was filled with anxiety and really wanted to cancel. But I plucked up the courage to go and I am so glad I did. Donna was the nicest person and put me at ease. I was introduced to seven other women and pretty much straight away I was as comfortable as I could be. The process of writing then boxing seemed weird, but as it turned out it was a perfect fit. I remember being so totally drained and exhausted after the group but eager to go back. And two years on I have no regrets.

Khale speaks...

Before these workshops, I had hardly ever spoken to anyone about the things that had happened to me. They seemed unspeakable. People don't like hearing these things. I had been silenced. Don't upset people. But mostly I was just so, so ashamed.

I still struggle with shame. It's not that simple. But there is a bigger feeling rising inside me, pushing my shame aside. I am angry. I am so furious at every sick fuck who ever dared to lay a hand on me or the people in this workshop or the millions of other people around the world who have been abused. I am angry, and I will not be silenced any more. I am speaking out. I don't care if it makes people uncomfortable. People need to hear this. You need to know that this is SO MANY PEOPLE'S story. These issues are RIFE in our communities, they are in our religious institutions, they are in our government, our schools, our families. It has GOT TO STOP. I will not be silent anymore.

Nikki speaks...

Before attending Left / Write // Hook, I'd already been in therapy of one form or another for 16 years. Each therapist and approach had been right at the time, but I'd increasingly been moving towards addressing my mind-body disconnection, and the fact that I held the trauma in ways I couldn't release through talking alone. I was constantly afraid. I knew that my default would be to freeze should I be threatened — but I had learnt to hide that behind smiles and humour. I felt the need not to burden those around me. I was taught that to be a burden was reprehensible.

Dove speaks...

Prior to Left / Write // Hook I had never attended any sort of group for survivors. I found the idea of speaking about my trauma in front of a group terrifying. I was overwhelmed by shame and feelings of disgust and isolation. I was sure it would just be another situation that would confirm I was an unlikeable freak.

Fortunately, this was not the case. I felt a great sense of pride at overcoming my fear and sharing openly and honestly, even though it was extremely terrifying and hard. I worked through some very heavy stuff during the workshops and felt relieved that I did not have to pretend to be fine. It was ok to be a wreck. The ongoing battles for me are deep feelings of shame and disgust (as it is for most survivors). Speaking out and being accepted really helped me. I am now able to be more open and honest about myself and my background in life and with friends. I can tell a diluted version of the truth now instead of desperately trying to think of lies to make myself look normal which often backfired as I'm a really bad liar.

The workshops helped me to feel less isolated and alone. Hearing the other women's stories made me realise what I feel, and experience is normal and common to many survivors. It helped me feel more accepting of myself. I now use writing more regularly as therapy and find it an effective way to communicate with my parts and give them a voice. I already used exercise as a strategy to cope with powerlessness, brokenness, anger, and rage. The workshops taught me to be better able to sit with pain, accept it and work through it. Boxing also makes me feel empowered and more able to protect myself in everyday life. Recovery is ongoing, I will never be well, but LWH has been a positive part of my healing.

Lauren speaks...

Before Left / Write // Hook I felt isolated. I lived a fragmented existence. I was able to present to myself and others as living a normal and functional life. My daily existence ebbed and flowed on a depressive spectrum, oscillating between feelings of total meaninglessness and a persistent sense of cynicism. I struggled to let go and worked incredibly hard, reaching for unattainable standards of perfection, and rarely letting myself rest. I had memories of what had happened, but they felt remote, disconnected. I'd come across stories from other survivors who looked and sounded like me, and I was starting to learn about trauma and its effect on the body. After close to 15 years of therapy I felt disillusioned and beaten down by the mental health system. I'd had a lot of fresh starts in my life, each time searching for an answer. I'd settle on something, only for problems to re-emerge or manifest in new ways. I now see that I was trying to find a new way of being that didn't feel so hard, while not feeling able to accept or admit just how hard I found life. It was a reality that caused me a lot of shame.

During

Julie speaks...

During Left / Write // Hook I wanted to give up so many times, but we had started the process of filming for a documentary. I didn't think twice about doing it as I wanted my story to be heard and to help other women out there who had also been silenced for so long. During this whole process with some help and support from my partner, my counsellor and LWH, I decided to report the crimes and finally let someone in authority know. This didn't happen overnight; it was something that had churned me up for such a long time. Once again, I was at PARC and with support, I made that phone call. It was the hardest thing I ever had to do. Anyway, I did it. I really believe I could not have done this if it wasn't for LWH. It gave me some power back. When Covid hit, we had just started filming and then it all stopped. We did our sessions via zoom and that felt totally weird. I felt disconnected from the group but still turned up each week. Finally, we went back at the end of the year. The other women are so supportive and kind. And without this process I don't think I would have achieved what I have today.

Claire speaks...

I felt held in the workshop space. I felt a sense of community and safety. I felt encouraged and supported emotionally, physically, mentally, and psychologically. This was because I knew I would not be judged or belittled. I felt safe to speak and write freely.

As I pushed myself physically, I felt strong, I sweated freely and felt free to go hard and exhaust myself. I vocalised as I hit the bag and accessed deep buried anger and felt safe to do so.

I had body memories and although it was terrible it also felt good to be real and be unmasking what had been hidden by decades of repression and societal silencing.

When I became emotional it increasingly felt more like release than overwhelm, it felt more manageable and real. When I had insights and realisations it felt strengthening and clarifying and less confusing or shameful. My mental and emotional state became one of focus and intention to be more truthful. I felt the environment of the workshop instigated and supported a strong sense of purpose and conviction. This sense of purpose and conviction has solidified in me to take into the rest of my life, the determination to support and encourage real and lasting change.

Lauren speaks...

In the first workshop, I felt very nervous and a deep sense of imposter syndrome, like I wasn't a *real* trauma survivor. I was overcome with emotion. It felt as if the extent of my suffering was recognised for the first time; a powerful affirmation that it wasn't all in my head. The weekly workshops became a container where I could exhale completely. If I felt shame, I said it. If I felt everyone in the group hated me, I said it. I challenged these feelings. The group held each other in a radical space of acceptance, love and understanding. We reminded each other of our resilience. We made space for each other. We wrote to prompts and learnt to trust the process. Hearing everyone's writing each week often triggered feelings of rage, disgust, hopelessness, hopefulness, shame, and sadness. These feelings rested in a powerful context of solidarity. This felt, and continues to feel, deeply political to me.

The physical practice that followed our writing challenged me every week. Boxing is hard. Every time I felt my body being pushed to its limit, I felt the bubbling up of shame and panic, the traumatised parts of me coming out to remind me I was weak, pathetic, that I didn't belong in the group, that my abuse wasn't bad enough to 'count.' But I kept going. Emerging from the other side of the boxing practice, I always experienced a shift. My experience varied from week to week, but through movement something always happened. It grounded me, and in a profound way it showed me that I can influence my experience by connecting with my body.

Dove speaks...

My experience of the workshops depended on what I was working through and what was happening in my life at the time. It was often an emotional rollercoaster; I was often surprised by what came up. At other times I was too shut down to connect with the workshop.

I always felt very anxious and exposed going into workshops. I felt I was *outing* myself as a survivor, even though I knew everyone was in the same boat, I found that very confronting. I had not had great experiences speaking out before and this was the first time I had attended any sort of group for survivors.

In time I learnt to let go during writing and allow my parts to express what they needed to; I was often surprised by what I wrote. The writing gave my parts a voice and a chance to be heard outside of a therapy setting. I was always nervous about sharing what I had written and worried about how others would react, but I was determined to do it and always glad I did. I struggled most when I was emotional. I hate showing weakness and vulnerability, even in a safe environment as it was never safe for me to do so in the past. After sharing I would feel relieved, no-one ever judged me. The other women would regularly express emotions, experiences and beliefs about themselves and the world like mine.

I have used exercise and boxing for years to cope with my trauma so was more comfortable with the boxing/workout part of the workshop. I did find it hard to let go during boxing and connect with my emotions be it deep pain, anger, or rage. I find it difficult to show these sides of myself as I have always had to keep them hidden. I had to make a concerted effort to sit with the emotions that had come up during the week/workshop and then focus them into the workout. Over time I became much better at this (though not always) and used it during my own workouts to work through everything from rage to feeling weak and powerless. I loved boxing with the other women. After sharing such personal writing, it made me feel like we were really connected and healing together. I really missed this connection during the online workshops. I found by the end of the workshops I always felt exhausted but also relaxed and grounded and proud of what I had achieved.

Khale speaks...

Before I attended these workshops, if you had asked me about anger, I would have said that I am not an angry person. I never get angry. It's just not part of who I am.

Every week I turned up, I wrote, I got deep into my own trauma, and I listened while other people shared. I heard so many heartbreaking stories week after week of the incredible evil that people are willing to inflict upon others. I so often felt so deeply sad and ashamed, sometimes to the point of tears, as we shared what we had been through. It was all just so completely unfair.

Once we transitioned into boxing, I found that something had been awakened in me. As we puffed, and grunted, and PUNCHED, I got angry. I was completely enraged. From the very first time I punched the bag, it was as though something snapped inside me that had been coiled tight for my whole life. I AM SO ANGRY. I punched and punched and punched, every week, getting angrier with every story we shared. I cannot believe how much anger I've been carrying around my whole life, never addressing. But now I know. And now I box. I get angry, I swear, I cry, and I punch until I am exhausted. It feels good to be this angry. We SHOULD be angry.

As I went through each workshop, I began supplementing the weekly workout regimen by doing my own exercise at home during lockdown. Throughout 2020 I went from a *couch potato* to a strong and fit person. I could run, I could do push ups, I could punch, I could lift weights. Slowly my body began to feel strong and hard. I was fast. I was strong. As someone who has spent so much of their life hiding inside afraid of the world, I can't tell you how different it was to navigate the world in this new body. I feel so much less afraid because I feel so capable. I know I can fight; I know I can run away. I have spent my life hating my body, but now I treasure it because I know it can protect me. I can protect myself. I didn't know it was possible to go for a walk outside without feeling terrified. I have been transformed.

Nikki speaks...

I do not think I will ever forget the visceral emotional and physical experience of the first workshop. It was the first time I had spoken to more than one person at a time about my abuse. Even in therapy I had been using euphemisms like "childhood trauma," I was never explicit. But in that first workshop I wrote about it. And it was so challenging to put the words to paper, and then to say them out loud. My throat was constricting, the tears were running, I could feel myself shaking. I had NAMED my abuser in public, and part of me was screaming that bad things would happen, that even though he's been dead for over a decade, that he was going to get me. To get us. And then... nothing happened. He didn't get us, and nothing bad happened.

I remember getting up and hitting the bag and feeling the emotions flow through me — I could see his face and I was hitting and screaming and vocalising everything I've kept inside for so, so long. And then my arms felt weak, and I heard the voices inside my head growing louder, reminding me that it was bad to fight back. The voices started to rise and try to make me be quiet again. I was shaking and crying, curling over on the floor, sobbing like I had never been able to before. And then there were arms around me, and someone whispering to me. Not to stop crying, or saying it was all going to be ok. I don't even think it was with words, but just knowing that for the first time, I felt like it was ok to feel this way, to react and to grieve. That the person holding me knew exactly what it was I was feeling, and that they were there with me, not taking it on themselves, but just holding me while I felt what I needed to. They weren't taking my load, my burden — they were just letting me put it down.

I left that day and felt empty in the most beautiful way. I'd released something I had forgotten I'd been holding. I went home and slept through the night. Even now I can still feel that hug — it gives me strength, and permission to feel.

After

Julie speaks...

After Left / Write // Hook I felt much stronger in my body and my mind. I still have a long way to go but I lost a lot of weight. I felt powerful in so many ways. Firstly, I went to the police and made a statement. Secondly, I have spoken out about my abuse and my mental health. If seeing me do it can encourage one other person, I will feel content. If I hadn't found Donna and LWH two years ago, I don't know where my life would be now. I say thank you out loud to everyone that has been through this process with me and to all the women in this group. Without love and support this group would not have worked.

Lauren speaks...

Left / Write // Hook was a structure of safety that held me through a transformative period of discovery and grief. I now have a language and a framework that I can use to understand my trauma. I have an improved sense of connection with the people in my life, with other survivors, and with myself. My sense of connection with my body has increased dramatically, and I can now notice when I disconnect. I still experience ongoing and at times profound grief and depression, as I continue the process of understanding the scope and impact of what happened to me and mourn for the life that I lost. I am trying to be kind to myself and sit with these feelings.

My idea of recovery changed while participating in LWH. I now recognise that it will be a lifelong journey. This made me feel very sad. I feel so angry at the injustice so many people suffer, at the violence of our systems of dominance and the complacency of our policy makers. But I also feel a renewed sense of agency, that recovery is possible. I intend to recover. There is no shame in surviving child sexual abuse. I reject your shame and put it back where it belongs.

Nikki speaks...

The workshops helped me to express my feelings and tell my story, but also to connect to my body. The workshops happened to be running in tandem with some deep work I had been doing with my therapist around identifying and connecting in with my *parts* of self, including my inner child. I talk a lot about her in my writings. The two — the therapy working to identify my needs, and LWH helping me to express and connect back to her and our body — have helped me immensely. I feel the last year has been one of healing. I'm not healed, and I don't think I ever will be. That's something I know in my heart and accept. But the workshops have helped me to connect and feel closer to myself and my history.

The workshops also taught me to identify what I was feeling, hold space for it, and to release it. I never felt bad for needing to stop — it was ok for me to stop. To rest. To listen and respond to what I needed in the moment was empowering. The ethos of the workshop was always about learning to identify and respect what each of us individually needed. It was ok if you needed to scream, or to cry, or to join a session to do the writing, and then do stretching or yoga instead of boxing that week. It was about what each of us needed. I know for me; my needs have never felt like a priority before.

I feel more ownership of myself than before — ownership of my body, my mind, my needs — my story.

Recently I was able to put all of this into practice when I was faced with a threatening situation. An old man I didn't know came up to me in the street and started screaming in my face that I should die. He was very persistent about it. He reminded me of my grandfather, my abuser. For the first time in my life, I didn't freeze. I kept walking. I walked away from him. I could do that for two reasons, firstly I was connected to my mind and body. I was able to stay in the moment and not switch to child mode. I was the adult, and I could protect myself. Secondly, I'd spent the last year learning to box, lifting weights and learning to be strong in my body. I suddenly realised he was old and weak, and if he tried to touch me, I could defend myself. I kept walking. I walked all the way home. I did what I couldn't do when I was a child and was so, so scared. I called the Police and told them what had happened. I protected myself, and my community and hopefully that man gets the help he so clearly needed. And after all of that, I let myself cry. I knew I was safe and allowed myself to feel it.

Gabrielle speaks...

Before Left / Write // Hook there was nobody to share my feelings with about my incest experience.

LWH was one of the best experiences of my life. I got to write about my incest in a different way for the first time. I could share with other women with similar experiences. I could express my anger in a healthy, positive, and grounded way through boxing.

Sometimes during Covid I took breaks from LWH because of my fatigue from my diabetes.

After LWH I missed it, but I felt more healed.

ROUND
ONE

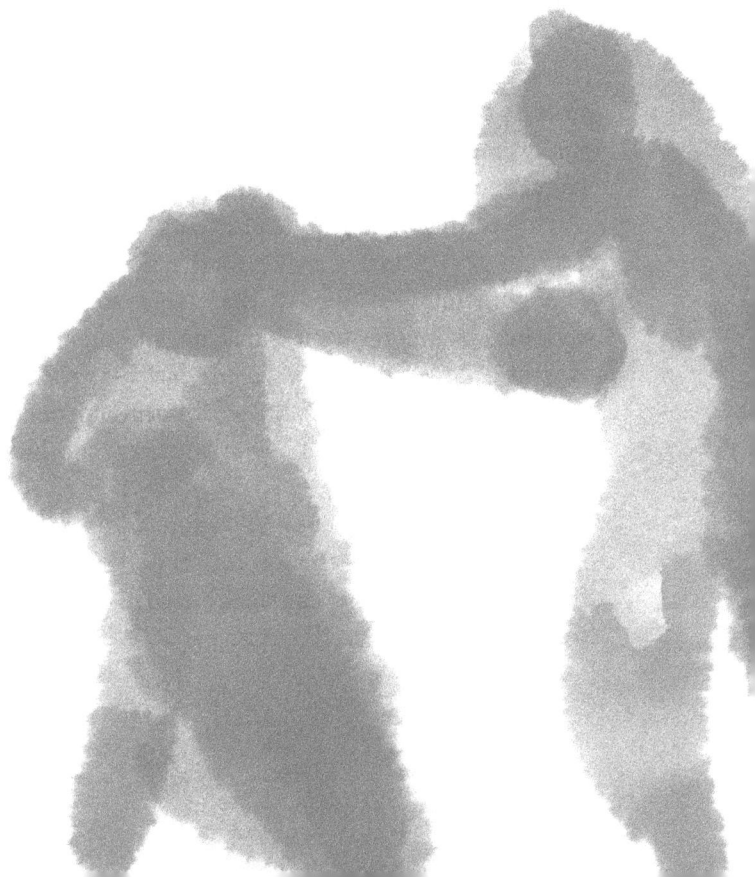

About Round One

Donna

The first hour of the workshops were spent using freewriting techniques (writing without self-censorship, to a given prompt). All prompts were purposefully focused on inviting participants to explore unconscious beliefs and thoughts about their trauma. I set the timer between 10–15 minutes. Then we shared our writings. The workshop guidelines state that although sharing is voluntary, it is encouraged, as the purpose of the workshop is to challenge the silence forced upon us as children. Every week, everybody shared, which helped to build mutual trust and community. We do not give feedback on writing, rather we thank each other after sharing.

Sometimes I would include a second prompt, setting the timer for two minutes. These short, pressure driven moments often produced surprisingly powerful pieces. In the second hour, the focus shifted to boxing, to give direction to the feelings and emotions that had been expressed.

The focus of the prompts in Round One were on identifying key characteristics, traits, feelings, and effects of our trauma. I chose these prompts simply because they were of most interest to me. Whilst some were purely creative, most of them spoke to what I had experienced since coming to reckon with the memories and impact of my childhood sexual abuse.

Due to the sudden turn of events with Covid-19 during Round One, some of the prompts spoke to the themes of a 'virus' and 'isolation.' The guidelines of the writing were to write continuously, without stopping. If anyone went blank or got stuck, the group were instructed to write the words; "*what I really want to say is, what I really want to say is...*" over and over again until a breakthrough occurred. These writings are not censored or edited. They are our raw and hidden truths, our creative and *temporary selves.*

The prompts are included before each poetry section so the reader can try their hand at them too. I hope that by unearthing your feelings, thoughts, and beliefs it can offer alternative insights into your sense of self to aid new and preferred narratives.

Round One Writing Prompts

I am here because | Being here

I connected and... | To punch is to...
Hand to cheek, I step, I punch, I...

There is no wonder | If it hadn't happened
Now that

The virus | My mother is a foot

Isolation | Madness

Vulnerability | Disgust | Shame

Mind | Body

I Remember | Being Believed Means

Recovery | Healing | Things I Like

Power | Fighting Back | Compassion

The last eight weeks

Choose one prompt at a time from each grouping above.
Turn your timer on for 10 minutes and write non-stop using
the prompt as your starter line.

I am here because | Being here

Claire

I am here because I want to save myself. I know I am here because I am sitting on an orange tub with pink wraps beside me. I am here because there are trees and I could walk in the forest. I can hear pens moving. I am here because I am hot and flushing and my glasses are fogging up. I am here sniffing. I am here because I was able to say it is them not me. Things are fucked, I am not fucked. I am here because I could pull a blanket over my head, a blanket of solitude, of safety. I am here because I could create a shield around me. I am here because I decided to be, to stop self-annihilating, to practice grounding disciplines. I am here because I could say I needed to change the people I had around me, not me. I am here because I can float around the ceiling. I am here because fuck it, it is time. It is safer now than thirty years ago. I am here because I want to feel real. I am here because I am angry and strong. I am here because I want community. I am sick of the isolation that saved me. I am sick of getting so locked in myself that it took some aggressive person to break me out of it because I was so far down the tunnel under the bed in the forest in the dark down the corridor that I couldn't get out. I'm here because of denial, denial gave me positivity enough to practice breathing, believe and hope. It wasn't denial. It was determination not to get beaten. But it was denial that saved me, not fucken remembering, but it also stole my life. There was no reality. I am here because I am going to face the pain of my original relationships, to stop repeating them, to stop feeling not real. I am here because I have a mask. I have a persona that can be presentable. That can pretend. I am here because I want to have a shared reality. Madness is not having my story. Not knowing my story. I am here to have a story, beginning, middle and end.

Lauren

I am here because I'm tired of being treated like there is something wrong with me. That I'm somehow deficient, damaged, not right, too much, intense. I'm sick of not being given dignity as someone experiencing the very real and well-documented impacts of trauma; an experience I had no control over. I am sick of having to hold this inside me and pretend it's not there to maintain my identities, as a professional, a friend, a family member, a student. It's part of my formation, and it's not going anywhere. So often I get responses from people that question my resilience. I get overwhelmed and stressed easily. I get sick often. I feel the weight of other people's trauma — people in my life or far away in other countries and contexts — as though it's inside me. My own struggle sometimes leads me to see the world as a cruel and heartless place, where people are constantly traumatised and re-traumatised, rejected and abandoned. I'm lucky because my story involves some of the best examples of support, care and love, and the people around me have not found it easy but have signed up for the journey with me. I don't have time for anyone who doesn't now. Since facing up to this, I've been much more open and matter of fact about my trauma. I don't share my vulnerability and struggle unless I'm with people I trust, but I'm starting to include it as part of the *facts of me* that I might share with people. Because by not acknowledging this very real thing that has and always will be with me, I'm self-silencing.

Donna

I am here because you silenced me. You choked me.
    You tried to break my neck.

I am here because you lied to me. You strangled me.
    You shoved lies down my throat.

I am here because you burned me. You handcuffed me.
    You spat in my face.

I am here because they fried me. Stabbed me. Poked me.
    Raped me. I am here.

I am here because you looked at me with ugly eyes.
    You called me a worthless piece of shit.

I am here because the sun went down. Chaos began
    and the bats flew overhead.

I am here because the sky went black. The clouds disappeared
    and I saw myself walk away.

I am here under duress — because your actions
    forced me to consider.

I am here because silence seeped through my veins. I cut them.

I am here. I am here. I am here.

I am here because danger hit the dancefloor.
    Neon lights circled me.

I shook the ground. I shook the ground.

I am here because of your depravity.

I am here because you tried to fucking kill me.

I am here because it rained and rained and rained.

I am here because I swam in mud. Drowning.

I am here because *what I really want to say is,*
what I really want to say is, what I really want to say is,
what I really want to say is…

I want to reclaim myself and I am embarrassed to say that because it sounds false and disingenuous and like I'm using buzz words, but I don't know how else to say I'm trying to put myself back in pieces, ripped up, chewed up, spat out pieces.

Every week. Every day. I am here because night-time brings terrors. Days bring disgust.

Each moment is a struggle with shame.

I am here because I want to dance with shame. No, deny it. It's your shame. It's your damn shame.

I am here because the lights went out and I crawled terrified in the dark to find comfort in a corner, so scared of the webs and I prayed and prayed and prayed for the light to magically turn on until I could soothe myself back to sleep. Shaking. Self-shaking. Disembodied me.

I am here because I am.

Gabrielle

I am here because

I felt like a bird on a barbed wire fence.

The same fence around the paddock my brother told me to turn toward. Then, when he told me to turn back, I saw the terror of his genitals.

The shrink said it's natural, its normal, children do that all the time. You show me yours; I'll show you mine.

Then why did I feel forced to show him mine?

Why did seeing my brother's genitals scare me so much?

Why, when I was deciding to obey and take off my clothes, did I feel terror?

He laid on top of me and stroked my sparse blonde pubic hair and said, 'you are becoming a woman.'

I react now as a woman by rarely having sex and by fearing sex, especially with men.

But maybe it is good I didn't have sex with the last man who actually wanted it because I didn't feel safe.

My body, my child self, my emotions are numb.

I feel like I have imposter syndrome, as a shrink and a social worker said my experience was minor.

But my current psych says it isn't.

Dove

I am here because my mouth is the only weapon I have left, they took everything else from me but never managed to shut me up.

I am here to empower myself and beat the shame that has followed me my entire life. To give a voice to myself and others like me. Too bad if you don't want to hear it. I lived it for 20 years.

I am here to overcome my fear of cameras, today is a big day for me. After years of child porn, I am facing a camera by choice for the first time and so far, holding it together.

I am here because so many have not wanted to know, found it too hard to listen to. People are outraged ritual abuse occurs in their own backyard. Victims are silenced.

I am here because boxing is empowering. I choose to be here, when to hit, when to fight. No ring drawn on the floor, no forced fights for spectators, losers are not gang raped or tortured, I am not being driven by fear.

I am learning to protect myself, de-program. I am allowed to say no and fight back against those who wish me harm.

This is me overcoming repressed memories and defying those who fractured and programmed a maze of parts, confident I'd never remember or tell. But I have.

Nikki

Being here today is an act of defiance. I belong, I exist
and I'm here to kick some fucking demons out of my head.

What I really want to say is a big fuck you to abusers and bullies
— to the old man on the train with a demeaning smile and love.

What I really want to say is I'm grateful to be here, and to see
the kind of strength shown. These women are superheroes,
survivors, or if you prefer, professional badasses.

I want to walk in the light without being afraid. I want to
know that I can defend myself, fight my own battles and
punch a guy in the head if I need to. I want to feel strong;
I want to feel safe — I want to be connected with my body
and soul. Today, I want to take that control.

What I really want to say is I want to be heard; I want to feel
ok about speaking out. I want to scream "fuck you" at his grave.
I'm scared at what will happen as a result of this process.

When did I learn shame? As a 9-year-old I wanted to shout
it from the hilltops — this happened to me and it was not ok,
it was not my fault. When did that change? When did I shift to
feeling the need to be silent? *What I really want to say is* I'm sorry
to the younger, inner me. I'm sorry you were failed by the adults
who were meant to protect you. I will make sure you are safe
now. And all at once I am her again, and I am afraid. I am so
tired of being afraid. I am so tired of being.

I am here because I want to exist — I want to take up space,
and not be some emotional sponge anymore. I want to know
my feelings and release them.

I want to fix my body and my mind and feel strong.

I want to feel strength radiate through me.

I connected and... | To punch is to...
Hand to cheek, I step, I punch, I...

Claire

I connected and there is the sound of traffic, in external veins. I connected and there is curled foetal and let the shoulders down like letting the curtains down on the stage, not in the public gaze. I connected and there is the rattle of a car going over a bridge, connecting this to this. I connected and there is a leaf from outside inside. All is inside, what is outside. Is there a line I can draw around myself to say I am, she is. I connected and sleep could absorb me like paper towel absorbs water. I connected and started sweating; wipe my forehead on my sleeve. I connected and I can feel the mat under my backside, my glasses fogging. I connected and what is it to not sleep. There is that crossing over where there is no connection. There is wakefulness, watchfulness, no connection to separate self, just the eyelidness of a statue, no letting go, no trusting. What happens to just being able to spill. It is not a boundary around self. It's a lack of connection to self, a frozen statue with no eyelids to close, behind closed eyelids, I can close, open into sleep, into not knowing what will happen, not being frozen awake in fear. I connected and there was a sense of stability, mobility, a sense of a border in a borderless landscape of sleep, not a control of what will come up, let go of planning for a possibility. I connected and I could feel a sense of being okay, of being in body. There was a time I could take off my clothes and swim at a waterhole, lie in the sun and sink into presence. What did it take to feel connected, to be separate, to not be other to self, to not be extinguished by a story that did not involve me? What is story, what is language, what is body, what is breath, what is being connected? I connected and I was not determined by someone else's story. I connected and I was independent, not dependent for my life, my survival on those that would do me harm, take my story and tell a story that I was not in. I connected and I felt it didn't matter;

I didn't need permission or approval to exist. I connected and it's about my own terms, being with others and being other together. Being I and we independent and interdependent, supported not suppressed, assert not overpower.

Be and respect other, there is a line in the lino, in the sound. There are foam squares and rusted 1kg weights in a crate.

Lauren

I connected and then collapsed. It's strange moving through your own life enduring the ricocheting effects of things from your own past, without even knowing. The connection is a revelation and a disaster. The world looks different now. I'm present, I'm here, I'm me, it all makes more sense. *What I'm really trying to say is* I can't unsee it now. I can't unsee the giant web of trauma that grows and shifts and hides beneath the surface. *What I'm really trying to say is* I'm fucking angry. I know how it happened now. I know the reality of a system that devalues and undermines and holds down and makes it all so hard that it only seems possible to give up. But I didn't give up. I guess that's something. I thought I was strong. I felt proud of the things I endured, the shame I moved through, the feelings of utter worthlessness that I didn't let overcome me. But the more I engage and connect, the more I feel held hostage by the brutality that surrounds me. I can't unsee. I'm so angry. *What I'm really trying to say is* I think I need a different strength now. I'm not sure what that looks like yet. The relentless and thankless work of women who surround me, as they courageously forge ahead despite everything working against them — it gives me strength. It doesn't feel like the word strength does it justice. What is it that drives us forward, despite everything? Why do I think it will get better? *What I'm really trying to say is*, I am, *what I'm really trying to say is not easy to say.* Love, truth, justice. These things are so real to me. Their reality is known to me. *What I'm really trying to say is* I'm sick of apologising for feeling things. For carrying the burden of knowing the total all-encompassing emptiness people are capable of experiencing; of knowing the grief of a life robbed from you; of knowing what it means to move through the world with less power, less agency, less opportunity. I know and I see and I feel and I express and I'm opinionated and I've lost count of the times this has got me into trouble.

Donna

I connected and I disconnected. I fell down a black hole, a spiral of darkness. It felt safe. I found out later it was dissociation. I connected and I laughed as though it was the most freeing experience, an unknown to be celebrated. I rolled on the floor. I cried.

I connected and I broke down. I shivered and shook, you held me in my arms as I became child. I was embarrassed.

I connected and I ran. I fled the room. I broke up with you. I left and it took days to come back.

To connect is to get hurt. A paradox because to connect is what I desire, is what I need to feel and move on, yet I sit scared in the corner, looking out through a long lens telescope, eyeing the situation.

Buried. Amnesic. Shake to the bitter end.

I connected and I thought I was going to die.

I had dreamt about it for so long, wished it, craved the release, yet to feel it, to feel the feelings seep through my body meant a nervous system exploding, a wailing, a deep cry from the Arctic, a sound so painful that writing it on paper hurts.

I connected and I froze.

I connected and I cried.

I laughed and I danced, and I took psychedelics and talked to trees. I humanised. I dehumanised. I raged. I buried my head under a blanket. I swallowed the truth for fear you would hate me, not believe me, ridicule me, throw me in jail, lock me up, blame me, hate me, you said you hate me. I was only little.

Why was I so bad?

Why was I so disgusting?

Why was I born so dirty?

I connected and prayed and then felt the shame writhing through me. I felt the shame seeping through my skin, staring back at me through the mirror. I couldn't quite see who I was.

Why I looked like that. Why was I so big? I was different than I had imagined. I once had a ponytail. Why did she cut it off?

It didn't matter what I did or wore or tried. Within hours a new feeling state embraced me. I connected and then I lost the line. I swore at myself in disgust. I angered at me for doing that — for being wrong.

I was programmed to hate myself. I connected and got fried. I connected and had pain through my abdomen. A silent existential pain — disconnected from me yet like an energetic force, it engulfed me. Keeping me from going insane. A silent friend. The disconnection. The despair. It saved me. It nurtured me to a bittersweet end. It clouded me like a warm blanket. It muffled my existence. It sang me lullabies, I so desperately wanted sung. It erased me from existence. Silent despair. I connected and then I forgot who or what I was connected to.

Gabrielle

To punch is to…

Imagine hitting the face of the man I went on an online date with who deleted my conversation thread because I wouldn't fuck him.

Who didn't really want to be friends who just wanted a fuck.

To punch is to…

Imagine my brother's impish face when I hit the punching bag.

To punch is to…

Imagine my brother's ex-girlfriend's face when I hit the punching bag. Because she tried to push her way into my flat. Who called me a *mad slut*. Who threatened to charge me with defamation.

To punch is to…

Imagine the faces of all the people when I hit the punching bag who say it is understandable that my brother would want to charge me with defamation.

To punch is to…

Imagine the faces of all the people when I hit the punching bag who say I am *really weird*.

To punch is to…

Imagine my ex-friend who told me I was *really weird*.

What I'm really trying to say is why did I stay friends with someone who put me down.

Dove

Hand to cheek, I step, I punch, I connect. She is backing away,
nearing the white line. I will win, I am stronger, there is no joy
in it.

I step back, I give her a moment, a judge is ready
with a cattle prod if she goes out of the line.

The crowd boos. Why have I stopped? *Sick fucks.*
They want me to finish her. There is terror in her eyes.
I allow her to regain her feet, I will be punished for this.

From behind I am shocked with a prod for showing mercy.
My knees buckle, the other girl is shoved forward. If she is going
to win this is her chance. I am kicked from behind, the girl takes
her chance, takes me down, sits astride me. She is the winner,
but she looks miserable, as do I, we both know the ordeal is far
from over.

The crowd is restless, their sadism not satisfied. I am stripped,
held down, the girl is handed an object. As victor she is
given first go and is expected to rape me. She tries to refuse.
Eventually the fear of what will happen to her if she displeases
them wins out. She takes the object, does as she is told, to
the cheer of the crowd. A judge yells at her "Harder! Do it
properly!" She complies while trying to apologize with her eyes.
I don't blame her, I try to let her know, then prepare myself for
what is still to come.

I don't know how they are selected but the men come forward
one at a time. They twist me this way and that. The crowd
cheers, especially at the sight of blood. The crueller, harsher
and more sadistic they are, the better.

I am raped, urinated on, sodomised and humiliated. When they
are done, I try to get up in defiance but have to be dragged off.

There is no wonder | If it hadn't happened Now that

Julie

There is no wonder I feel like a train wreck

I try to hold my head up high but I almost crack my neck

If only the world could see what really happened to me

I wish I was made of glass and maybe my torture would pass

How can one be treated with anger and neglect

Will my story ever be told I don't know but I'll have no regrets

When I was a child I had a horrible time

So much abuse and torture I want so much just to die

I was taken every day and discarded by the way,
    no wonder I was so absent

I really didn't want to function

There is no wonder I felt I have no future

Only coldness and such a lack of kindness

When you think one torture had ended

Another pops up and takes you unaware of what's
    around the corner

My days are now filled with horror and nightmares

I battle the voices that haunt me in the darkness.

I get judged way before people know the real me

And they define me with an illness without seeing within

I know I am all scattered and my mind is in pieces

But I try every day to fill in the blanks

Only to look at you and see even more cracks

I want to speak out and let the world know

Just who I am but I have so far to go,
   I feel so abandoned and worthless within

I want to scream and shout and don't let those bastards win

I'll go through the court with my head held high

And hope they'll be taken down and rot till they die

It will never be over but it won't be in vain

I won't let anyone else go through this pain,
   I went to the roof to just end it all

But in my mind did I really want to fall

My voices took over and I lost sense of time

Only to be looked at and judged all the time

Khale

There is no wonder I am always afraid. I've always been afraid. Even before I could remember being hurt, I was afraid. I was a child who didn't like to be touched. My mum would joke that hugging me was like hugging a brick wall. She said the same thing about my cousin. It made me wonder what else we had in common. By the time I was a teenager and started to socialise at church, people noticed I didn't hug anyone. I just didn't like the way it felt. Like being trapped. Having no control. I always needed to be able to get away. I hated being held. People say that hugs make them feel safe, but they feel like a prison to me. I have since learned that a hug can feel safe and reassuring, only if it comes from someone who I know won't hurt me. It takes a long time to get to that point. There are only two people in the world I like to hug. Still, I'm glad I have learned why people like it.

There is no wonder that mum always said I hated men. Even before I remembered the abuse, I always hated men. It was easy when I was little. You could complain about *boy germs* and people would think it was normal. But when I was big enough to have breasts and hips and all those other horrible things, people wouldn't accept that line anymore. "Why don't you like boys?" "Are you a dyke?" I didn't have a good answer anymore. I tried to hide behind religion, saying I was saving myself for marriage. But that wasn't true. I just didn't like men. I don't like the way they smell, how they talk, they laugh — every word out of their mouths seems like an attack. Maybe because I was so small for so long. Inside every grown man I can't help but see an enormous potential for violence. They are too big. They take up too much space. They are too loud, their bodies too hard. I hate the way they feel when they press against you. The weight of their bodies is too much. My body was always just too small. Men are so heavy. Their hands are so big. Their breath is too hot, their mouths too wet. It's no wonder I always felt so scared. A man's body will overwhelm all your senses until you can't even breathe. I nearly choked from the bed sheets, but my ears and nose and skin were flooded with everything else. Everything male. Half the world is men. It's no wonder I'm always afraid.

Nikki

There is no wonder I am drawn to the type of sports
that hurt me. There is no wonder my body betrays me.

There is no wonder my mind fragmented and broke.

I feel responsible and disconnected. My body, my mind
and soul were separated and still struggle to reassemble.

I didn't say anything — I didn't protect those around
me and I felt I deserved to break. But it's not my fault —
a reality I struggle to accept.

The more I push it away the more I break.

Is this all in my head or is it some kind of bullshit cosmic
punishment? That can't be it — it would be the ultimate
unfairness to punish a child for being raped and then
manipulated into saying nothing for years.

That would be some old bullshit.

I'm afraid of the phantoms my mind creates and paranoia fuels.
The presence in the dark made real by memory and experience.
The ever-present fear, constantly reaffirmed by day-to-day
interactions.

What I really want to say is I'm sorry.
To the others I didn't protect.

What I really want to say is I'm sorry.

What I really want to say

What I really want to say is I'm drawn to the only contact position
on the field in an effort to re-enact the protection I couldn't give
those seven little girls whose lives were also destroyed. I couldn't
protect them, but here on this field I might be able to stop this
goal and help these women.

Is that stupid? Writing it out makes it feel that way —
the realisation that it doesn't make sense.

None of it.

What I really want to say is I'm so sorry to the child inside, that you had to bear that weight. That you were abused and lied to. *What I really want to say is* it wasn't your fault. It was his. He was an adult; you were a child — and he lied. He said if you were silent no one else would be hurt — and he lied.

You deserved better, and he deserved to burn.

You deserved better, and he deserved to burn.

What I really want to say is

What I really want to say is

What I really want to say is

What I really want to say is boxing provides a release.

What I really want to say is your body isn't betraying you, but you need to listen to it.

What I really want to say is that you need to be present.

What I really want to say is

What I really want to say is you're not broken yet.

What I really want to say is

What I really want to say is stay with me in this reality — don't go to that place that borders on memories in flesh.

Claire

If it hadn't happened? I can't imagine what it would be like if it hadn't happened. I wouldn't be crashing against rocks all the time. I wouldn't be dissociative. Can I even imagine how I would be if it hadn't happened. I wouldn't struggle with intimate relationships. I wouldn't be shaking when I touch what happened, even dipping my toe into the mass of red lava. If it hadn't happened I would not be here with this group. Traumatized people are my tribe of reality of tents pitched by a flowing river. If it hadn't happened I wouldn't need to understand it's not the relationship. I'm projecting onto it, the thing itself, the thing that's happened. If it hadn't happened I wouldn't be the person that has to try every day just to be. What happens when your home page, the place where you were formed, the place I was formed was the place that denied me form? If it hadn't happened I could feel for just one moment I was safe. If it hadn't happened I could live, not fight through veils every day. If it hadn't happened I could hear the bird and hear the bird not say to myself I am hearing a fuckin bird and someone mowing. If it hadn't happened I would belong to reality, not have to practice fucking belonging to reality, grounding and whatever other fucking healing modalities just to have an experience of fucking feeling human. Just one fucking day free of dissociation. Couldn't I go on a cruise ship, a holiday from having to believe every day I am in this body, I deserve this existence. Denial or depression, dissociation or excruciating pain, what a fucken choice. If it hadn't happened I wouldn't think I am going to get hit every time a man expresses a feeling that they are upset. I wouldn't go into, if I don't fix this I'm done for. If it hadn't happened I wouldn't have to try to be all the time. I would just be. I wouldn't have to carry the leaden boulder of pretending I'm alright just to function every day. I wouldn't have to pull myself back, watch myself pull myself back, it's not happening now, you feel like it's happening now, but it's not happening now, fucken self-talk. If it hadn't happened, I could have one day of life breathing freely, not having to remind myself to breathe. If it hadn't happened I would not be with this group of women silently together. That's in my heart like a bird not broken with all those tiny bones that come together in flight not fright, in flight not fright, if it hadn't happened.

Lauren

If it hadn't happened I wouldn't have spent my life reacting, coping, excavating just to move forward. *What I'm really trying to say is* it feels like such a waste. All the things I ever dreamed of doing or changing or creating always come second to my trauma. They are pushed down, made harder by it. If it hadn't happened maybe I would have enjoyed the freedom of being young, instead of feeling trapped in myself, alone in my pain. If it hadn't happened maybe I would have liked myself more, spoken up more, felt more. *What I'm really trying to say is* I'm exhausted. All the time. Living is exhausting. I can't remember a time when it wasn't. Actually that's a lie, because I do remember. I had a spirit. I was a force. Energetic, excited, I ran before I could walk. That changed. I became *the one with issues.* There's always one with *issues* right? If it hadn't happened maybe I would have lived a totally different life. *What I'm really trying to say is* it terrifies me to think about what my life might have been if it hadn't happened. It feels like all the blood moves through me in waves, a nausea I can't escape. The sadness of what could have been, the regret. The shame and the anger. If it hadn't happened maybe my first sexual experience would have been mine to choose, the beginning of a healthy exploration of an empowered sexuality. Maybe I wouldn't have believed that empowered sexuality meant sex with anyone, proving that I'm desirable and wanted. Maybe I wouldn't have let a man 24 years my senior convince me I was his equal at the age of 19. Maybe I wouldn't have always needed an older man's approval. If it hadn't happened I might have energy for things that matter to me that are just too hard. I might not have fucked up multiple friendships with emotional outbursts, gaining a reputation as being *highly-strung* and *emotionally fraught.* Maybe I wouldn't have formed my identity with the idea that I was fatally flawed, damaged, wrong. Maybe I would have played sports. My body has always been a site of anxiety and fear. It wasn't mine to own or control or love. It was mine to fix and hide and make smaller and less. If it hadn't happened maybe I wouldn't have got cancer, but I know this is not true. It just seems cruel, why beat me when I'm already down. You put me in that cupboard, I don't remember how, but I'm only just re-emerging.

Gabrielle

If it hadn't happened...

I would not have had a nervous breakdown.

If it hadn't happened...

I would not have been locked up in a mental institution.

If it hadn't happened

I would not have been so triggered that I became *insane*, *unwell* or whatever the feeling is.

There is a lot of stigma not only about mental illness but also about Graylands (the hardcore mental institution in Western Australia).

A so-called friend judged me because I was institutionalized in Graylands.

He asked me if I was put in Graylands and I said, "I forgot I had" and he said, "you would want to forget."

When I was in Graylands I ordered pizza from inside and when the pizza parlour asked my address and when I said Graylands, they hung up the phone.

Getting counselling about incest the first time really spaced me out and placed so much stress on me that I became mentally unwell.

But in this writing workshop I don't feel like that. I don't feel unwell or very triggered. I don't feel like the world is going to explode.

If it hadn't happened...

If my brother didn't sexually abuse me, I might be able to have a sexual relationship. I might be able to have sex because I wouldn't feel so scared.

What I really want to say is...

If it hadn't happened...

It would not have brought tension on my family.

My father who is now dead seemed to be on my brother's side when he said my brother, "had no recollection." I remember when I was last unwell at the university trying to tell people that I was an incest survivor, but they just saw me as mad.

The student support officer at the university said not to tell people at reception that I was sexually abused as a child because they just saw me as the mad lady.

Khale

If it hadn't happened, I probably would have thought that it was OK to go to parties. I probably would have felt that sometimes guys are just nice to you because they want to be friends. Because they think you're cool or something.

If it hadn't happened, I wouldn't feel so ashamed of my reactions. When I see someone that looks like him, I cross to the other side of the street. What do people think of me when I do that?

If it hadn't happened, I wonder how long I could have lived before learning what corrective rape was. But I did learn. He explained it to me. The reason I had to follow all of his directions, quietly — because there were three of them, you see, and if he alerted the other two, then they would all teach me together. Better my being gay be our little secret, and he could deal with me, here, quietly, in the dark, where it is impossible to escape because this van is going 80km/h.

He definitely taught me something that night. For better or worse, I learned that I could override my dissociative state. I could feel myself starting to black out as he held me down, but I knew that if I did, it would be so much worse. So, I forced myself to stay present, to stay in my body, to feel everything. To feel where every part of him was. Every point of contact.

What I really want to say is, even though I got away after he threatened to kill me, did I really get away? If these are the scars I kept, if I still carry these memories and still relive them every time someone whispers in my ear, did I really survive?

I remember thinking when he invited me to that party, that maybe not all men are bad. Some are just friendly and nice. And maybe that's true. But it's a pretty big coincidence that my first ever excursion with a man in the lead turned out this way.

Maybe I really was just naïve.

Maybe I should have known better.

But I thought I did everything right. He was a co-worker
I'd known for a year. I knew where the party was, but that
turned out to be a lie. I knew some other girls who were going,
but that turned out to be a lie too. I didn't drink. I tried to find
some women to cling to. But when it came down to staying
in the house of a man who had already tried to jump me,
or getting into that van with him and the others...

Did I make the wrong choice?

What choice did I have?

I tried to be safe.

I don't think safety was an option that night.

Julie

Now that the decision is made my heart feels lost and empty

I know what is right but nothing feels right
Just like that day on that fateful night
I just left work with not a care in sight
I cashed up the till and locked all the doors
Not realising I was followed down the long corridor

I slowly walked to my car and out of the blue
A stranger had followed all masked and in blue
I was pushed to the ground and a hand on my face
I couldn't scream or get out of that place

I lay there lifeless and the next thing I know

My skirt was taken from way down below

I grimaced with pain

And then time passed me by

The rocks in my back hurt so much I wanted to die

Finally it was over and I just couldn't move

I looked for my keys but they weren't to be found

I scurried along the dirt on the ground

I got into my car

And just sat there in horror

What just happened

My thoughts triggered one another

I don't remember driving home but when I finally did

I showered until my skin just bled

All I could smell was a scent of meat

Do I go to the police or sit there and freeze

My mind was fractured and my body was lifeless

Do I tell someone or do I just sit in silence

Eventually the time came to go to the police

They fobbed me off

To deal with my grief

He's still walking free and I really hope what happened to me

Won't happen again to anybody else

In this time and space my world is shattered

But I'll pick up the pieces

And hopefully I know this pain will lessen

And my heart will flow

What I really want to say is...

Nikki

Now that we have connected, we can see our experiences reflected back at us. For me this brings a comfort that I didn't know I needed. To know someone else implicitly understands. *What I really want to say is* I'm both angry that it happened to any of us, to anyone at all. But I still find a comfort in you all.

What I really want to say is I'm tired of reliving a waking nightmare. Of feeling hands that aren't there. I'm tired of feeling unsafe in a world that keeps reinforcing that it <u>is unsafe</u>.

What I really want to say is

What I really want to say is

What I really want to say is I want to fall asleep without being afraid and I want to wake up without being scared of a new day.

What I really want to say is that being locked in brings me comfort — for me the greater fear is being forced to go somewhere I'll be trapped.

Right now — in this room I can feel the extent of me, and the walls bring comfort. My ability to lock out the danger brings safety. A door that's shut by me is power.

What I fear is being forced to go back and be locked in a house by someone else, by him. To see my parent's car retreating down the dirt track and feeling his hand on my shoulder and knowing there's no one to protect me — that I can't protect myself and there's nothing but the expanse around me. Even if I run there's no way and nowhere that will be safe.

What I really want to say is I don't want to keep reliving this.

What I really want to say is I want to feel safe in an expanse — to be able to feel safe alone in the world. Instead of just in this room with a locked door — looking out at a world that we should all be able to feel safe in.

What I really want to say is now that

What I really want to say is I don't fear this pandemic as much as I fear being trapped with an old man. I don't fear this virus as much.

What I really want to say is

What I really want to say is I'm alone feeling safer
than surrounded by a crowd.

What I really want to say is a big fuck you to the people who make
this world feel less safe — to the drunk men who block the paths
and yell obscenities. I wish that just for a moment you could
be this afraid of the dark and the monsters like you that haunt
it. For one moment to look in a mirror and for them to feel
the terror and horror and disgust their actions inspire.

The virus | My mother is a foot

Donna

The virus was in me, shot through my veins. I drank the virus
years ago. Poison bleeding out of my pores. The virus was
suburban home, melancholic mind, isolation. The virus soothed
me, placed me in strangers' bedrooms, plastered me to walls,
kicked shoes in my faces. Stared at me through the mirror,
rubbed itself over my body.

The virus was bred into me from an early age.
It disintegrated relationships, it swam at the bottom of the pool,
it spoke to me late at night. It whispered my name.
It hypnotised me. It sang lullabies.

It cracked open my door and beckoned me out slowly.
It sang in the dark. It danced in my dreams.
The virus said "die." The virus said, "I hate you."

The virus said, "you filthy slut, you dirtbag."

The virus stank.

The virus ate.

The virus lay dehydrated by the toilet bowl.

The virus was a fragment that covered my face,
held open a smile so you wouldn't know it lived inside me.

The virus coaxed me to the dark recesses of my mind.

The virus caught my tongue. Held it tight, clamped shut,
so no words could come out.

The virus made me breathless, it stripped my mind.
I could no longer see in pictures.

I lived in the richness of my imagination. Worlds built,
so incredible, so lustrous. Full of riches and gold and
trinkets that would dazzle you. The virus stopped
me from remembering. It caused lights to flicker
and distant distractions.

The virus. The virus. The fucking virus.

I see it on the washing line. It's in my clothes. It's in my hair.
I feel it clinging to my ears.

The stench is so bad. It's rotten to the core.

It smells like burnt liquid, cake, I threw up the virus, it said
it was gone, but it came back. Night after night, day after day,
week after week, month after month, year after year, it grew
in concrete, it lived in my sheets. It showered with me, between
my toes. It dated me. It had sex with me. It kissed me. It stroked
my face. It was so gentle with me. I gagged silently — sickening
— it tasted so sweet — it told me it loved me. The virus married
me. It had my babies. It decimated me. It created new selves
to have new relationships with. It dated me multiple times,
each time it said it was going to be different. Each time it said,
"trust me," "believe me," "this time it will be different,"
but it was always the same.

The virus drove me in circles, fast, the virus covered me in
blankets. The virus said, "hello, be my friend." The virus said,
"don't talk about me." The virus said it was all my fault.

Dove

The virus frustrates me, it brings out the best and worst
in people and has started to show me things about myself.

The virus shows me how selfish people can be, obsessed
not only with self-preservation but with profiting from it.
I loathe and am disgusted by them.

The virus highlights how many horrifically stupid people
and how many malicious people are out there.

Thankfully, the virus also highlights the good, beautiful,
generous, loving people. I thank God for them.

The virus makes me feel angry and combative. I have spent
my entire life terrified of some of the most evil monsters
imaginable and survived them. I refuse to be afraid of it.

The virus has shown me just how afraid of death people are
and how little I care. I have experienced far worse than death
many times over and I don't fear it. What surprises me is how
much I welcome it, to be able to stop fighting, to finally find
peace, escape the pain, fear and torment. Escape my painful,
damaged body, the memories, nightmares and flashbacks.

The virus has shown me how desperate I am to be free.

What I really want to say is, I am tired and worn out. I have had
enough; I don't care about the idiot virus and won't hide from it.

What I really want to say is, I am hurting, feel unable to cope,
I can't take this virus on as well. I don't have the energy; I have
to put it aside. My head is already full up of memories in need
of processing.

What I really want to say is too ugly to write. *What I really want
to say is* full of anger and hate, hurt and pain. I am unable to put
it to paper.

What I really want to say is, I want the world and its virus
to fuck off.

Donna

My mother is a foot. She steps on me to bring me tea.
My mother is a foot. Long, odd shaped, angular, weird.
She despised me. No, no, she didn't despise me, she loved
me in uncharacteristic ways. She served. She did everything
a mother should do, except develop a relationship with me.
Not that I need a relationship with her, or do I? It is a luxury
for some. The Mother's Day commercials suggest we should
have connections beyond servitude, but I never had that.
She was a woman who talked in tongues, strange verses,
statements that were matter of fact, based on nothing,
only the nightly news or a framework that was Catholic;
black and white, where I was destined to go to hell.

I dreamt of her, from a distance. I searched for her in a crowd,
eventually I caught up and she turned around and it wasn't her,
it was a woman who filled me with fear and terror, shaking to
my core. Teeth chatter. Chatter.

My mother is a witch, funny eyes, pointed teeth.
    She knew black magic and drank potions.

My mother goes to Church. Works in charity shops,
    bakes cake, has no bank account.

My mother serves my father. Cooks and cleans, like Cinderella.

My mother is a crazy... foot... standing on my neck, cutting
off my circulation, rubbing hands over strangers. She dines,
eats meat with her hands. Sits at the table last. Pours tea leaves
in the garden. Dances with us, awkwardly, looks sad, empty,
confused.

I got drunk and slurred and talked crazy. She said,
    "you sound like your mother."

I don't know my mother.

I don't think or feel or care or talk or wonder about my mother.
She is an abstract word — a noun — an entity with annual
celebrations — with breast cancer — with weird sayings
with black coats, with shoe boxes, with shoes in the cupboard
for each day of the week. With busyness, with distraction,
with shallow feet, with short, short hair, with cold, dark
eyes, clammy hands, on shifting sands. My mother is a foot,
standing on my head, stopping me from moving, until I see her,
feel her, taste her, mock her, push her, away.

My mother talks about the weather and writes me letters to
tell me she cares. Pragmatically, until I am crossed off the list.
My mother is a foot that walks over alters.

Isolation | Madness

Lauren

Have I ever not been isolated? I feel like I'm quite good at this. For my whole life I have felt separated from those around me. Different, maybe in good and bad ways. Like other people just don't get me or I don't get them. Like I was on a different trajectory. And in many ways, I was. I lost my sense of belonging so early, and I responded by bunkering down, committing to my own reality, focusing on what I could control. I became a *straight-A* student. I played the role of the talented, smart, passionate kid who could never just relax. But really, I was trapped. I held myself inside those standards of perfection because it made me feel safe, but what motivated me to keep going was my deeply held fear of failure, of giving in to my patheticness, of exposing how disgusting and wrong and damaged I was. My eating disorder was one of the calmest periods of my teenage years. A time of fixed and singular focus, of bettering myself and rejecting all imperfections, of perfect control and precision. It felt safe. I can feel it now. The memories are so strong. But then I lost control. I no longer felt safe. And everyone else was out of reach. I was alone in a desert, with nothing and no one to reach out to, and disappearing more with each passing day. Ironically, my fear of disappearing completely, and failing, was what motivated me to call it a problem, and crawl my way back up to higher ground. The two years following this moment were a blurry, scary, confrontational struggle. I felt like a newborn who had no natural sense of anything anymore. And I felt alone, so alone. I started doing therapy. Therapists are amazing, and I am so grateful for them. But I hated them too. I hated that they were the only people who knew, and I hated how they exposed me to myself. But through exposure I have healed a great deal. After high school my need for control morphed and changed and translated into different forms, mostly without me knowing at all.

Gabrielle

I kept singing the Sex Pistols like I couldn't stop. I bought "Never Mind the Bollocks" for the first time, although very late and I was addicted. They saw me as a danger to the community, so they put me in a hard-core institution: Graylands. I was in a locked ward. I couldn't leave. I was isolated.

Oh Graylands.

I thought I'd never get to the other side of you.

Oh Graylands.

I thought I'd never be free from you.

Oh Graylands.

I thought I'd never escape you.

I thought I would never live again.

But I do, I do live again.

I still have my life.

Now there is the isolation of lockdown, but it is not as bad as the isolation of Graylands.

I have suffered worse than this lockdown believe it or not.

My favourite song by Joy Division is called "Isolation."

I remember a terrified woman in the locked ward in Graylands how she crawled along the floor singing out, "let me out, let me out!" How she knocked on the door of the locked ward, singing out, "let me out, let me out!"

Khale

I have had so many periods of isolation in my life. None like this, I suppose — most I did to myself. But certainly periods of intense loneliness, of being cut off.

I remember when my first partner and I started living together. How suddenly I wasn't allowed to leave the apartment for anything other than work. How that space shrunk as she grew to fill it. How each day got angrier and angrier, my freedoms less. I couldn't call my family. I couldn't use the computer. Losing control of my finances. How my self-esteem dropped lower with every word she said to me.

By the time things got violent, I was convinced I deserved it. By the time the sexual abuse started, I thought that that was all my body was good for — let her have a go, get it out, get mad, cover my mouth and pin down my arms and just get it out until she was calm again.

My body could defuse her anger. I wish I hadn't learned to do that, but maybe at later times it saved me.

I remember after she finally left, I was free, but I hated myself so much that all I would do was get drunk and throw myself at the apartment walls trying to feel something. I locked myself away for so long because I felt so ugly.

I'm worried that being locked away now, those feelings will come back. I notice I want to drink more often. I look at myself with less compassion. I am so disappointed in myself for losing my ability to run and run.

What I'm really trying to say is, I'm terrified to find out who I will have become when we emerge on the other side of this. What if my mental health can't weather this storm? How will I survive without all the myriad things I usually do just to maintain myself?

Choosing to hide inside is one thing. I've done it many times. But being forced in is another. I'm so worried about what behaviours I might revisit the longer I am in this head space.

Julie

Madness… just what does that mean

My head is filled with darkness and despair

I feel like I am going nowhere

Sometimes my head feels so afraid

I just want to lay back and die

All of my voices just rant and rave

Somebody please dig me a grave

I search for answers with nothing in sight

All I want is to sleep all night

I know I can function to some degree

But my head's a mess and my body just screams

I can't stop shaking and my voices are intrusive

When will this horror end nobody knows

I'll just take each day and see how it goes

Madness engulfs me and spins me right around

Do I want to see around the corner

I'm scared of the madness that enters my head

I want to be free and let the light shine on me

Nikki

I feel the madness creeping up on me, beckoning, calling,
seducing. Accept it and disassociate for a while, be free
of the fear and maelstrom inside.

The madness speaks in a voice late at night. The madness
is at once a friend and foe. A lie and an ultimate truth.
It is real and it has passed.

The madness tells me that the world outside is unsafe, and that
people will hurt and lie to you. The madness is a truth and is
hard to deny when life and experience reinforce its message.

This week I had a therapy session and it allowed me to connect
with inner-me, the child who had been abused. She was
so afraid — afraid of the world and all around. She didn't
speak, she could not speak. All she could do was cower in a
corner and howl in silence and be silenced. She had been torn
and was so terrified that she could not accept compassion
or kindness. All she could do was cower, and howl silently
into her hands and be silenced.

She was so deep I couldn't reach her. It took guidance
to identify what she needed — she was so shut down.

What I really want to say is I was ashamed I couldn't help
her unassisted. It is so hard to be vulnerable after everything.
It's hard to be vulnerable when the option to be vulnerable
has been taken away at an early age. And all she could do
was cower and howl silently into her hands and be silenced.

I find it difficult to leave the house because outside is unsafe.
I fear leaving this relatively safe corner of the world and going
out into the world. At least this is known. So maybe I'll stay
in the corner and learn how to howl out loud and be heard
and not be silenced again.

What I really want to say

What I really want to say is

What I really want to say is maybe.

Vulnerability | Disgust | Shame

Claire

My vulnerability has been made public. I am silently screaming in a fishbowl, seen from the street. The wind is on the outside, the pen is on the inside. My skin is off. I am a pool of water a fountain rises from and falls back into breaking the sky the clouds into fragments. My vulnerability has gone public. The world is experiencing violations, zoom meetings are being bombed. We were so quick to stay connected. Driven by the mantra, stay connected, adjust, keep connected. The zoom book launch was bombed, out in the rain, friends faces fuzzy, the network not keeping up with the movement. The wall permeable, her smiling face unaware the chat was being bombed. I lose something every day. The government doesn't own the beach, define my relationships. Partners living in separate houses can or cannot visit each other. Vulnerable to government interference. No one questions married couples seeing each other. Relationships vulnerable to government definitions. Single women living alone can't isolate with one friend without being in a relationship. Why do single women living alone have to be more isolated than everyone else? Fuck that, they may have one single woman friend that they don't identify as being in a relationship with but in reality rely on like a life partner. Other countries are in stage four. What will stage four mean to my vulnerabilities. Vulnerability is the norm. I have spent a life building bridges that can be taken down. Between inside and outside here and there, this side and that side, public and private. I have a public meeting in a private space. I can have it in bed if I want. Vulnerability to vulnerability. Vulnerability is a vast open space, it's a space I can meet people in. No walls, no requirements. Vulnerability is a vast open space, an openness. Vulnerability to joblessness to homelessness, but not friendlessness. Vulnerability, if everything is online we are very vulnerable, politically and personally.

So reliant on it, what if someone pulled the plug, tripped over the cord. We have all taken the stickers off the camera we were so determined to protect ourselves from. I have ripped the band-aid off the camera, that camera that is that one eye pointed at the space between my eyes. It allows me to see but it sees me. That is vulnerability, what is vulnerability, being seen. Vulnerability is being seen. What is being seen by other? I get to see myself. I have to look at my fucken face while I look at the faces of others. I have to be present to looking out at me looking back at me, rearranging my face in the gaze that gazes back at me. It is my gaze I am vulnerable to. My gaze, gaze at myself, present in the video conference to be seen. People are leaving their blinds open to be seen.

Julie

I feel so vulnerable lying here alone

I step outside and wish I was a drone

I put my trust in some people's hand

Only to be dealt with misfortune and their demands

I feel the world doesn't understand

With a label of schizophrenia

They hear the word and everyone flips out

I'm not an alien and I don't have two heads

I am an individual who is vulnerable

From the trauma within

My heart is full of love to share

But when they see the word

They just sit there and stare

If only they knew how my world is each day

Never knowing which voices will haunt me all day

I wish I could tell how my childhood really was

All the abuse and trauma I endured

Now all they do is pop me with pills

But that's not what I want

I just need to vent and breathe

So much has come up and I don't know where to start

But someday I really need to listen to my heart

There are few people in my life

That know the real me

I can let my guard down and see the real me

I just want to cry and let it all out

Now I'm in lockdown and there is no way out

I wish I could tell the so called professionals

Just to get fucked and listen to what's within

Dove

Nakedness and vulnerability go hand in hand for me, I hate them both. To be naked is to be vulnerable. Vulnerable to violation, abuse, and humiliation. Each of the thousands of rapes involved me being naked and vulnerable. Whether ordered to remove my clothes, or they were removed for me, my nakedness resulted in pain, humiliation, and shame.

I particularly hate nakedness and water because a whole new level of pain and fear was achieved by my father or the group in a shower, bath, or pool. A favourite for them was my head held underwater or my mouth being held open under the spray while they took turns. The evidence washed down the drain.

To be naked feels vulnerable. I am terrified people can see what was done, that I am dirty, shameful, filth, only useful as a plaything. I had to keep my body a certain way or I was punished. I was programmed to perform naked, shameful, disgusting. It must show.

I hate my nakedness. I have to see the body I so despise, the used-up shell, all its flaws and ugliness. To see my body triggers memories of what was done to it.

Early programming was that it was my purpose to please men, it's God's will. As I was so naughty, I had to be punished at the same time. They told me I'm wicked then made sure I was.

What I really want to say is, I never want to be naked and vulnerable again, with anyone.

Lauren

Disgust, shame, silence. The dangerous trifecta. Sometimes I think silence is the biggest killer. It's the enabler of the shame and the feeder of disgust. I remember how viscerally I disgusted myself as a young teenager. I remember a chaotic night aged 13 or 14 when I turned up at my mother's bedside, wailing, inconsolable, pleading for an escape or an answer. "I hate myself, Mum. All I know is I hate myself and I don't know what to do." That pre-empted my decision to lose weight. I had no idea what was really driving this disgust. Neither did Mum. But it manifested most strongly when my body failed to meet expectations, when I couldn't quite get it to do what I wanted. School P.E. (physical education) classes brought such intense feelings of anxiety and shame. Any school swimming event was enough for me to question my whole worth. I guess it made sense to my teenage brain that changing and controlling my body would set me free, would allow me to see my true potential, and discover a version of myself that I didn't find repulsive. I know how that turned out though. *What I'm really trying to say is* I wasn't really there. My body was not mine. And it became less mine. I'd learned to only value it as a means for other people's pleasure and approval and validation. At the end of the day, I still hated it. I traded my love for my body for a sense of control. But did I ever have that love? I don't know. *What I'm really trying to say is* my body continued to fail me. My abuse set a blueprint. It morphed and got sick and writhed in pain and shame and sadness, inflamed and angry and overworked and underworked, overfed, and underfed, reactive not responsive. I tested my body's bounds, let men use it and abuse it and proved to myself that it was nothing, I was nothing. *What I'm really trying to say is*, I'm 27 years old and I feel like I'm only 'coming in' to my body now. I can see this pattern now. My trauma had a pattern of manifesting physically. The longer I continued to ignore it, the more the symptoms would manifest, keeping me in the cycle of disgust and shame. Silence bound this ritual together. Without silence it would fall apart. But then there's breaking silence in a world that does not want to hear it. A new shame.

Relationships challenged; indignities endured. Health systems that minimise your pain. Legal systems that maximise it. People who don't try to understand, don't see how resilient you are just to keep showing up at the starting line. What I'm really trying to say is it's fucking unfair. I keep waiting for a moment when the penny will drop, but I don't think it will ever come.

Donna

Dear Disgust,

I don't particularly want to talk to you. I hate
you. You hate me. Should we just settle on that?
Every day you permeate my existence. I wake with you.
You travel with me through the day, you put me to sleep at night.

You caress my body, rubbing it with sticky oil. I fear you.

Disgust, when did you first appear?

When I was a child, innocent flesh; you defiled me.

You pissed on me, covered me in red, you shoved my face
in dirt and buried me. You pressed on my body for hours.
I could not breathe. Your dirty breath.

Disgust. Get off me. Get away from me. I don't want you as
a friend, a companion, an enemy. I want clean sheets and to not
feel guilty after I have eaten or had sex or done something nice
or gotten dressed or glanced at myself in the mirror.

Disgust, you roll me in wet soot, you lavish me with your shame.

Shame of existing. I have a right.

Shame of my being. It's safe to be.

Shame of my body. I am strong.

Shame of my mouth. You defiled me.

Shame of my thinking. You programmed me.

Shame of my words. You silenced me.

I've been carrying you around since I was born.

An empty shell.

A heavy suitcase inside me.

Geometric shapes filled with horror stories.

I washed myself on so many occasions. It made things worse.

Sometimes I think I have been reset but the web weaves again
and I lay paralysed on another level.

Sometimes I think I have been reset. I lay paralysed
at another level.

Who pushes buttons?

Who controls the shame?

I've wanted to dialogue with you for so long.
I'm scared to hear from you. I'm tired of you. I'm over you.

"Make friends with the depression," they say.
"Make friends with the anxiety," they say.

How do I make friends with something that tries to push
me down — makes me feel less than? Diminishes me?

Why should I make friends with you? What have you got
to teach me? You are like them. A toxic waste dump that lives
inside of me. Threatens me. Hates me. Saddens me. Disgust.
I clean you up. I make you clean. I transform you. I show you.

Julie

Disgust and shame what are these words
It's how I feel and the torment really hurts
How dare those bastards do that to me
It was meant to be a game I counted past three
All the laughter but so much despair
My body's not mine

It was all those boys who thought sex was just fine
Every day I had no words
I didn't understand what happened to that little girl
Apart from the torment a nickname was used
I thought it was cool to be a part of that school

Only in time I started to see people would call out my name
But it wasn't what I thought they said to me
I thought it was horse because I was so tall
Only to realise that whore was the word
My body was taken every single day
For a whole two years I prayed they would stop
It became just normal but so very wrong
I felt out of my body as I watched from above

Disgust, Shame and sadness it was too hard to discuss
I was so young and I didn't really know
Any of these feelings will they ever go
To this day the flashbacks are real
I get in the shower and I just want to scream

I wash so hard my skin starts to bleed
Just to be rid of the odour that never does leave
I am starting to learn about my feelings inside
And process my thoughts very slowly but right

It was so long ago
But the disgust is still there
Maybe one day the pain will ease
Just by talking and letting myself breathe

Khale

I could write about shame for days. It is the central theme of my life. I am so ashamed of every part of my mind, body, and spirit.

The first time a psychologist asked me if I had always been ashamed, I had to think so far back. As a child, as soon as I could talk, they taught us: you are bad. You are a sinner. You were born with the devil in you, and you need to be washed clean from sin by god's love. Once I was a teenager, they started teaching me how dirty I was because of my body. A woman's body, with breasts and hips, even when my mind was still only 15. But women's bodies are sinful. They lead otherwise good men into acts of sin.

I am so, so ashamed.

I feel like every different thing that happened is another bucket of black tar poured over me, which I can never get clean of. These experiences cling to me like stains. I feel discoloured, filthy, so dirty dirty dirty.

The church taught me that bad things don't happen to good Christian girls, only to temptresses. Jezebels. Did I tempt each and every one of them? With my 23-year-old body, all skin and bones? With my 14-year-old body, just acne scars and braces? With my tiny toddler body, rolls of baby fat and still wetting the bed?

I am so ashamed.

I wish I hadn't gone so far backwards. These days I can't enjoy sex without feeling ashamed for days afterwards. Only whores enjoy sex. Only perverts have homosexual sex. I am so dirty, so wrong and sinful. I can never get clean.

I know in my logical brain that it's not my fault. I'm not sinful. But when they tell you that — "You were asking for it. This is what you want isn't it, you little slut. I know you're just a horny little slut begging for it" — they keep telling you these things, and the preachers are telling you that it's your fault for having this body that breeds lust — how do you not believe it? What choice do I have but to feel ashamed?

It's my fault. It's all my fault. I never should have been born, and then I wouldn't have made sinners out of good people with my awful body. I am so ashamed.

I wish I could get clean, but I can't. I feel like I've been writing about shame my whole life. It's the biggest feeling I have. I'm sorry, I'm sorry, I'm sorry. I wish I hadn't brought my awful sinful body into so many peoples' lives.

Dove

Shame is with me every day, it's a part of me and has been since I was three and my father and his mates taught me the art of the blow job. I didn't know what was happening, but even then, I knew it was bad, disgusting and shameful.

It continued, being used as a tool to ensure my silence as I was continually groomed. Until, at the age of seven I was presented to the judgers, and the shame and humiliation rose to a whole new level. A panel of men led by an older woman. They were God's judges. I had been bad, wicked, naughty. They could punish me, and no-one needed to know. What if my mother found out and left in disgust, left me and my brothers with my father.

Stripped naked, I wanted to die of shame while penises and objects were put everywhere possible, and my body contorted into unnatural, painful positions. Afterwards, I would be shamed for any mess made, disgusted, and sickened by what had happened, I was told what a filthy, disgusting girl I was and dragged off to be cleaned up. Shame ensured my silence until dissociation occurred and they were free to do as they pleased.

The torture and rape sessions intensifying, made to feel ashamed of any reactions or attempts at defiance or escape.

Then the rituals started, stripped naked in front of large groups of adults, tied to an altar, forced to watch sacrifices, and perform for them with other girls.

Then came the prostitution, a new form of humiliation and shame. From nine, drugged, locked in a dingy room, while one revolting old fuck after another came in. Wanting to die each time the woman came in to clean up the mess.

Nikki

I feel like the shame has become part of the fabric of me.
It's woven into my story — like a single rotting thread through
a tapestry. The shame makes me doubt my worth — I exist only
to assist and help others. And if I can't do that — then what is
the point of me?

I feel ashamed of what I've allowed to happen —
to me and to others. I am shame.

I'm ashamed of my weakness, my uselessness in the face of
abuse. In my mind I imagine myself breaking down the walls,
breaking the faces of my abuser. But instead, every time I freeze,
I am frozen and disgusted at it. I am shame.

I feel ashamed of my fear — this virus reinforcing the madness
inside. Don't go outside — you'll catch the virus and infect all
those around you. It will be your fault and you'll be worse than
useless. It's the same message that used to ensure my silence —
if you tell anyone I'll be sent away. You don't want that do you?
You don't want to cause me harm? You have to stay silent.

Well fuck you. Fuck you and your manipulation, old man.

What I really want to say

What I really want to say is that my Grandfather would have been
in the danger zone for this virus — and he was a virus. He could
only survive off crushing and manipulating healthy cells — pure
young children. He could only survive off others, just like a virus
can't survive without a host.

What I really want to say is the shame is there but now obscured
by shaking of fear and rage. I've said it out loud, I can't take it
and he'll be mad.

The child inside screams in silent terror, while the adult yells out
loud through tears of rage — you fucker! This isn't my shame
to carry — it's yours. The knowledge is a vaccine, but not as
effective without acceptance of its reality.

What I really want to say is the line of reality is blurring
as I write this — the flashback and memory bleeds through.
Once I couldn't have stopped it — but now I can hold it apart
enough to function. Sometimes no one even notices that behind
the smile, the ultimate moat — there is a remembered voice
and hands. I guess that's the thing about viruses and shame —
even if you kill it, it remains there — dead or dormant.

Mind | Body

Lauren

My mind is my body is my mind is my body. My brain remembers and reconnects and plays out the pattern. The pattern is part of my makeup. It is now me. *What I'm really trying to say is* I am forever changed. When I was 18, I first admitted to myself — or realised, one of those — that what had happened was probably more of an event than I had previously thought. It's funny how I could connect with that notion but have no inkling that the traumatic teenage years I was emerging from might also have their origins in that *event/non-event thing*. Whatever it was I didn't know. I've seen psychologists, I thought. I knew this might have had an impact. I'll nip it in the bud. It didn't really mean anything. I went in thinking I was already fine. This is preventative. This is proactive. This is what the difference is between a victim and a non-victim. This will mean the weird pangs that appear in my gut and pelvis and shoulder and neck and eyes, every time this memory visits me won't happen anymore. I look back and wonder how the therapist didn't push me further, didn't help me see the connections between this *event/non-event/did-it-even-happen* thing and the pain and difficulty that had become my life's companion. All the issues or problems or patterns or mechanisms of my brain expunging this, she was helping me deal with. How could she not see? Or maybe she could see that I couldn't see. Did that mean I wasn't ready to see? Were my eyes seeing what my body wanted me to see? Was my mind holding what I wanted to hold? While I was setting out to protect myself from this abstract monster was it at work within me? *What I'm trying to say is* I was a child. I was a child. I didn't feel like a child. I always felt beyond my years, a few rungs removed from my peers, somehow out of reach from them.

Sometimes I felt damaged. Other times I felt intelligent or mature. I always felt alone. I assumed I understood myself, my hardship, my hardness. I just feel the world deeply. I just feel it all because I care. I feel it all, how can that be wrong? But it gets me in trouble. How can they not understand? How can I be in this place, having these thoughts, making these choices?

Donna

Body. I keep you strong. I like when you are frail. I wish you weren't here. Body disrupted, interrupted, I still want to hurt you, push you, disembody you. I run so you hurt, I keep thin, so I don't feel you. The worst is when I see you and feel you. I would prefer to be waif — pants fall off — little girl clothes. I am uncomfortable being an adult. When you look at me. I am afraid of your touch. Seeing flesh. Folds.

My mind is a puzzle.

I dissociated when I read about systems thinking, the complexity of my mind... the laneways. The maze, the web, the networks. Dismantled. Mind. Body. Body. Mind. Body as object. I identify with the object as one, within me. I separated so long ago. I was selves inside me, one whole. Many parts. The abstraction of self was not a mystery. I understood multiplicities, fragmentations, assemblages, lines. I drew the body as stick figures. Uncomfortable to give it form, as if filling in the lines would make it real. I remained geometric. Squares inside boxes inside triangles, stored on shelves. I was an archive. Uncatalogued. I was messy papers, cut up, found in the bottom of the drawer. The body seen from afar, viewed with shame, embarrassment. Wonder.

I wouldn't look at you this way. I would never look at you this way. I remain intrigued, with self, I refuse the mystery. Cut off. Difficult to breathe in the body.

We had face masks. To wear for shopping. I put it on, it was tight around my face, it pulled out my ears. I breathed in and felt their hands around my face. I ripped it off. "I can't wear this," I said. It was a memory.

I go blank so quickly. I wipe the slate so quickly.
I say yes and forget so quickly.

I could sleep for a hundred years. I would be happy
to wake when it is over.

I could sleep for a thousand years. I would be happy to wake
in another time or place or country.

My mind is so clear. I erupt with laughter.

My body is so free.

My mind is a maze of dis-connections.

Wires.

Spark plugs.

Worn shoes.

Worn smiles.

Worn eyes.

Worn.

My body.

Gabrielle

My body feels vulnerable.

My body feels powerless.

I keep putting on weight.

Growing fatter and fatter.

I have to be more disciplined with what I eat.

I have to exercise more but I feel exhausted.

My body feels out of control as it gets bigger and bigger.

Kathy Acker saw body building as a movement toward death.
    I see boxing as a movement toward life.

My whole body comes alive when I box.

I release anger in the most grounded way.

One of the reasons I put on weight was a reaction
    to my medication.

My medication causes my weight gain so I cannot help it.

People abuse me in the street because I am overweight.
    They do not realise that I cannot help it.

That it is because of my medication.

It is often other women who abuse me in the street for being
    overweight. They say "yuck."

When people abuse me in the street, I imagine shooting them
    with my imaginary bazooka.

Julie

My mind is my own

Even though at times I am unsure

It feels like I'm living a dream

With big bits missing in between

I try to think hard

And make everything right

Only to be pulled down

My body so tight

I remember the day

That my voices came

After all the abuse

Were they my saviours

While falling from grace

I thought they were my friends

And sometimes they pulled me through

Only to find out

They were bastards too

They fill my mind

With obscenities and demands

I would always listen

But try to step back

My mind sometimes feels

That it's not my own

I go through so many battlefields

Not knowing which way to go

I hate every one of them

But I am starting to see

One day they will leave me

And I hope to be free

Nobody understands how frightening this is

Sometimes I listen and do what they say

They have caused me so much grief

And tried to kill me from within

It makes it so hard

When your mind is so full

Those fucking voices need to leave

And not be understood

How do I explain to people

Who don't really know

They think I am mad

And put me away

Fill me with tablets

And then walk away

These voices don't define the person I am

There is so much more to me

Please take time to understand

Just sit there and listen

To my story I have told

Don't shock me with treatment

And all will be well

In this day and age

Compassion is right

Khale

My body is the source of all the problems. I didn't ask for this body. I didn't ask to have all the parts that apparently make me a target, or the high voice that makes me weak, or the gender that dictates that I'm supposed to be submissive.

I tried to save myself from this body. I tried to make it disappear. I stopped eating, feeling more in control the more my body ached. I started to disappear. My breasts dropped, my bum fell away, my hips shrank. People started saying "Is she OK? She looks unwell," "She needs to eat something," "She looks like a skeleton," but that was so, so much better than the catcalls and the gropes in dark places.

My body became so small, and frail, and smelly and hairy. No one would want me now. There was so much power in starving myself. I would run until I fainted. Finally, I was in control. No one could do anything to my body that was worse than what I was doing to myself. You can't stop me. I could cut myself into pieces and that would be my choice. This is my pain, inflicted on my body, by me, not someone else. Finally, my body felt like my own. I still hated it, but it was mine.

It all fell apart when I learned how weak I had become in that tiny frail body. It was so easy for people to pick me up and put me where they wanted — in that bed, or that car, or on that couch. I was so easy to pin down. My tiny arms and legs were so weak. All I had was my voice — that stupid feminine voice, saying no, no, don't, please stop, so politely, please don't.

My body was so tiny it was completely useless to me.

I want to be different now. I don't want to be small anymore. I want to take up space, I want to be strong, not from starving myself but from fighting. I want to be able to run without fainting. I want to be able to punch and have it leave a mark. I want people to think twice before trying to put me somewhere. I want the pain I inflict on myself to be the pain of progress, of growing, of breaking out of that old small body with the tiny voice.

I want to shout. I want to swear. I want to be loud and angry. Girls aren't supposed to be angry, but we have the most to be angry about. I want to be angry for all of us, but especially for me. I want to take up so much space that people get out of the way. I want people to be too scared to even think about touching me.

I want to be strong.

Nikki

My body is a vessel for my soul, a canvas that others project feelings, desires and judgment upon.

From my perspective I do not love my body, but neither do I hate her. She is a meat sack — something that holds my essence. Society tells me I should love my curves, hate the images projected upon it.

This body is the medium through which I experience and interact with this world. It's how I've experienced being abused, but also intense love — the comfort of my lover's embrace.

What I really want to say is my body is part of me, but it is not my entirety.

The times I've hated my body it was due to others projections and actions — the memory of them imprinted on flesh and made part of my story. The experience is written across it — see here is where he grabbed me and forced me down. Here is where a man on a public bus put his hand down my top and grabbed my breast — and the bystanders did nothing.

Here is where another man grabbed and pinned my shoulders to the bench and licked my neck and face on a train platform at peak hour — and 100 bystanders did nothing.

Here is my experience of an unsafe, untrustworthy world written in flesh — read my story and then tell me straight faced that I should trust more — that the world is safe. Lie to me. But I won't believe you — the story written across my body reminds me — makes me relive the feelings, the touches, the fear.

What I really want to say is I am lucky to have as balanced a view of my body as I do. I love her some days — my hair, my eyes. It's a place where I can be safe — or at least that is the eventual goal. I don't always have to love — despite the pressure to. This is a meat sack I inhabit, and that is fine. If you don't agree — that's your problem, not mine.

My value as a person, from my perspective at least, has never been tied to my body. Others may do that — I remember having my belly fat pinched and hearing her say "oh you would be so skinny if it wasn't for this bit." The pain of the pinch and the words stay with me — even now I can feel her finger grabbing, words cutting. But those were her issues, her concerns, not mine. This is my meat sack, and it is fine the way it is. It's my vessel and my connection to the world.

I Remember | Being Believed Means

Julie

I remember when it first began

I always remember I ran and ran

What was I escaping from

And where did it lead

Always down the same old path

With nowhere in between

Trees were all around me

And the sounds of birds were there

But only in my dark world

Was horror and despair

Did anybody know what was happening to me

Crouched down with torment

I always wet myself with fear

When I was found

It all began again

Not just one

But five older men

How could they want to torment a child

Is that why, I became so wild

I didn't understand

I thought there was something wrong with me

When I wanted to play

With kids in the street

They always said no

I was knocked down with defeat

I thought the only way

For me to be part

Was to have sex with each one of them

But I knew it was wrong in my heart

I remember I always went through life

Always thinking somebody wanted to take parts of my life

I even thought in my late teenage years

I might as well do this always

And get paid in return

I would push people away

And never get too close

Afraid of being hurt, or rejected or worse

I remember the day

Eva came into my life

She made me feel giddy

But I didn't need to pay a price

I only told her after a few years

What happened to me

I was scared she would blame me

But instead she just gave me

So much love and compassion

To this day

She is my one and only companion

Dove

I remember too much, what I don't, my parts do. I remember how I changed from a chatty, intelligent, curious little girl into a dissociative shell in survival mode. I have been this way ever since.

I remember withdrawing, the light going out from the world, it became dark and scary. I could not cope. I remember wondering what was wrong with me, why I couldn't fit in, why everything was so much harder for me. Why was I such a disappointment? So fundamentally flawed? Why couldn't I just be normal? I remember being desperate to be normal.

I remember the blackouts, a world filled with pain and fear, where I was told I was just a hypochondriac and drama queen. I remember terror every time I had a shower or went to bed. Would he come tonight?

I remember developing, being disgusted by my body, being informed I was a woman now, time to please men. I remember being disgusted by the mess that meant I had pleased them. I remember telling my dad I was pregnant at 12, how he blamed me, called me a slut, and wanted to know why I wasn't on the pill. That he now had to fix my little problem. I remember feeling filthy, ashamed, confused.

I remember no longer being able to cope with school, with being around my peers. I remember the pain, self-loathing and hatred, disgust, and shame. I remember the beginning of my eating disorder and the first time I picked up a blade. Feeling release and relief as I watched the blood flowing down the drain, like I had created a valve to release the pressure.

I remember being so overwhelmed with pain, I couldn't take it, I wished desperately to die and make it stop.

Lauren

Being believed means being a trusted witness to my own experience. Being believed is loving myself enough to honour my worth. *What I'm really trying to say is* being believed helps me find "me." Most of my life I feel like I have constructed my identity from my perceptions of everyone around me.

Gabrielle

Being believed by my current psychologist

helps me heal,

as the other

psychiatrist and social worker

invalidated me.

They said my experience was minor

compared to other patients.

They said I should just forget about it.

Julie

Being believed means I have taken back some power

It means I can finally feel freer

Being believed means someone's finally listening

And acting on my words

With force and control

One day justice will behold

Khale

Being believed means my story is real. That it happened, happened to me. That it's OK that I am so far behind everyone else because I had so much more to overcome. Being believed means not being told to be quiet, to never mention such horrible things. Being believed means being accepted, it means so much, it means I am OK.

Dove

Being believed means everything. It means validation.

Nothing is more devastating than being told your experiences don't exist; SRA (satanic ritual abuse) doesn't happen, repressed memories and DID (dissociative identity disorder) are false. This denial empowers perpetrators.

Recovery | Healing | Things I Like

Claire

Recovery is a distant country across brown water with no technology and old boats to get to it. Recovery is what the fuck do I need to recover from. I've always been this way, what is wrong with the way I am. This is my reality. It may be under weighted blankets of clouded sky but this is my reality. I have a problem going to big shopping centres. I don't like fluorescent lights and long corridors and mazes and can't find the toilet. I don't like being manipulated to walk through the store to find the escalator. This is not something I need to recover from, shopping centres are fucked, with stars hanging on fishing-line to disorientate me. Recovery is the smell of grass, not what is going round and around in my head. It is the moth plastered to the outside of the window, wings spread to the light bulb moon. Recovery is recovery to myself not some abstract idea of normalcy and a distant country I do not have a passport to travel to. Recovery like an island in the middle of a body of water. I am the body of water not the island. Recovery is hearing the waves gently lap on rocks and the passing police boat and him saying you are going to get wet when the wake makes it here, splashed sitting on that rock and me not caring watching the wake form a wave coming towards me and watching it approach and feeling the setting sun on my face and chest and sitting in the wake of the setting sun. And tying ribbons to wrought iron gates, gates of churches. I had been collecting ribbons from flowers students had given me, pinning them to the corkboard in my kitchen. I didn't know why I was collecting those ribbons. Recovery is saying the way I am is normal. Being in the kitchen on the floor not being able to move is a normal response to a murderer getting off. My sister likes it when I get angry. "I can't," she said.

She has to stay stable, she says. "The medication is working," she says. Yes, working to keep her head under water blowing bubbles of smoke in the face of endless days in front of the table she used to dance on, paint pictures on. All the colours, the colours of cloaks. She stood at the door. She read me all of *The Magic Faraway Tree*. Fuck recovery. Recovery of what, recovery of memories. Recovery of lost keys. Recovery from the flu. Recovery from being hungry every day of my childhood. Recovery of her sight. Recovery of motherhood. Recovery of sanity. What is recovery.

Gabrielle

For some reason I cannot write about positive things like recovery, healing, and the things I like.

The first thing I thought about for *things I like* was McDonald's, which is pretty bad.

Believe it or not I rarely eat McDonald's. But I bought McDonald's to eat yesterday to treat myself because I had to sit a really hard test at Uni.

Things I like. I like the Left /Write // Hook workshops because I can relate to the other women. I can try to understand my overwhelming emotions that are destructive, like how I had a suicidal thought a week or so ago.

I remember my childhood.

My brother placing a dead mouse in the palm of my hand.

And how upset I felt that the mouse was dead while my brother registered nothing.

Now I try to think of something I like.

I like my new book, it has a beautiful cover. I am so glad my publisher accepted me. I did a radio interview on a queer radio show for my book.

The queer radio show was really cool, it was called *Pride and Prejudice.*

Khale

Recovery is such a shitshow. For most of my adulthood when I've thought about recovery it's been about eating disorder stuff. Or self-harm. My big secrets that I was constantly trying to hide. The recovery journey from a physical addiction is so much easier to map. Two steps forward, one step back. Good days, bad days. I don't tend to think of healing from trauma as a recovery journey. Maybe I should. Carrying around all these assaults like a bag of rocks, and every time I think I've taken one out — I've dealt with that, processed it, cried, let it go, moved on — but then not long afterwards I get triggered again and I realise my bag is still full of rocks.

I remember every time. I remember every sensation in my body. I remember every word he or she said, or if they didn't speak at all.

What I'm really trying to say is, what does healing look like? Does it mean forgetting? Or just not caring?

Sometimes I don't want to remember any more, like that would be easier. But I need the lessons I learned. Don't get in cars with boys, even friends. Don't get drunk, even with girls. Don't get into relationships with people who are too broken. Beg to sleep in bed with mum instead of in your grown-up bed all alone in the dark.

Don't, don't, don't.

Don't be too friendly. Don't be too noticeable. Don't be too understanding. Don't be small. Don't be naïve. Just don't go anywhere or do anything or trust anyone.

I've had so many discussions with my partner about learning to trust people. To accept that some people are good and would never hurt you. But you just can't know. You can't know who would betray you if they had the opportunity. It's better to never take the chance.

It feels like such a childish emotional state to be trapped in, the space of not trusting. Feels like I need to grow up. And I am trying. I go to therapy, I take my meds, I put in the work. But I'm not sure that I want to become a trusting person. That just sounds like being a target again, and I want to be done with that. I want to believe that last time was the last time. That I'll never have to look in the mirror and see myself covered in bruises again.

Lauren

Healing is being honest. *What I'm really trying to say is* pretending as if everything is normal, there's nothing worth noting and it's too much to confront, is no longer an option. Like I can't win if I put myself up against it. Because acknowledging the pain and beginning to heal also requires you to accept the future. The growing pain. But mostly all the ingrained ways of being that are your homeostasis, that can't be changed as soon as you decide you want to heal, confront, or move forward from. It's still there holding you in its survival grip. *What I'm really trying to say is* healing isn't easy. It's a hard choice. But I reached a point where not-healing was harder. It seemed unfair. No moment of magic or therapist or friend or relationship or meditation practice or running regime or spiritual reflection changes the facts you are working with. They have a role; they push us forward — I take that back. Why do I find myself always reaching for *productivity-speak*? As though my healing is some sort of KPI (key performance indicator) for my life's success. Since deciding I would confront this, my concept of healing has frequently shifted and changed. It's a hard slog. Structure keeps me sane and helps me feel safe, but my need for rigidity also makes me feel unsafe. My sense of safety is exposed as superficial. Feeling safe isn't about certainty. It's taken me a long time to learn that. Nothing is certain. You can't control what happens. I lose my sense of safety when my body and mind spiral and I feel powerless to stop it, like my own brain is waiting for me to have a weak moment so that it can strike. *What I'm really trying to say is* it's another lie. It's another version of the shame and self-destruction and self-disgust. I have a belief that my own body wants to cause me pain. My mind has an agenda to unravel me. It's so hard not to feel powerless in those moments. It takes so much energy and courage and feels utterly painful to resist the urge to fall in a heap and declare I can't go on anymore. Maybe I need to resist less. Maybe I need to just be honest, sit with it, feel it. I'm learning. Each time I get lost I study it, analyse, and reflect, forensically examine why it happened.

This is my survival brain at work. But I didn't know that even six months ago so maybe I'm one step closer to knowing what to do? Every now and then I have a day, afternoon, evening, or hour of feeling total peace and calm, buoyed by my own strength, my unending resilience. I feel proud of my voice, my story, my life. I feel thankful and joyful and alive. I feel responsive and observant and interested. These are the moments I'm always reaching for. I have faith they are getting more frequent, like an inner compass. I will believe. I will keep going.

Nikki

Healing is slow, one step forward, two steps back. Sometimes healing is pushing a boulder up a hill. Sometimes it's being brave in the dark. Sometimes it's being brave enough to stop and let settle.

It's not a linear, or an easy process. But it's worth it for those moments when I realise the progress that's been made. Like the moment I could let myself be comfortable and intimate with another person. It's knowing I can fall asleep, and they will be there when I wake up.

Healing is difficult. I will always remember a counsellor describing it to me like this —

> "The pain and the memories won't get weaker
>   — but you will get stronger."

Sometimes healing is an unpleasant truth. It's knowing that the road ahead is difficult, and long. Sometimes healing feels a lot like failure — because as I beat one part, one symptom, one aspect another changes. Sometimes it feels like fighting a damn hydra — lop off one head and another grows.

To me — sometimes healing is fighting like a boxer in a ring saying stay the fuck away. This is my space, and these are my boundaries — respect them. Other times it's naming the beast and then sitting with it as the storm crests and falls. Sometimes it's the strength to remain soft and kind when a world's worth of experience tells me to become hard and cruel. Healing is knowing when to fight, and when not to.

What I really want to say is that I guess healing, the ultimate state of being healed, would be to feel safe to be vulnerable. Vulnerable and Safe.

Healing feels like sleeping in a warm cloud, loving hands rubbing my back — and knowing that this love is true, and this space we have built is safe and beautiful.

Healing is all of it. And the road is worth it. As a favourite lyric of mine said "if the end is worthless, we don't need the journey." This is worth the fight — the end and the journey both.

Donna

Healing is a big wound you dress for me.

Healing is cups of tea I refuse to have.

Healing is self-soothing crap I read in privileged magazines.

Healing is throwing rocks at my window and remembering
shards of glass.

Healing is sweet, soft angelic breath, washing blood off
my body.

Healing is running my body against cold, hard gravel and
begging, begging for you to wipe it off. Healing is the truth.

Gabrielle

Healing.

My mother said, "So, it's opened up a can of worms."

That can of worms made me end up in a mental institution.

I dreamt that my mother and brother were driving me in a car.

And they kicked me out of the car.

Dumped me.

Julie

Things I like are very simple

I love my wife and the colour purple

The things I like always comes from a heart

Always together and never to part

I like the way my head feels on my pillow

I also like to stand under a willow

I like to play with Charlie each day

Khale

I like it when she kisses me gently. I like that she always asks my permission. I like that she stops if I get quiet. I like that she holds me until I calm down. I like that when I apologise for crying and making my face ugly (like mum used to say), she calls me beautiful. I like that she looks at me as though I have nothing to be ashamed of. I like that I can still feel this way, even though I am so broken.

Dove

Things I like. Sounds simple, easy, everyone knows what they like. Except me. I am weird, a freak. A product of a lifetime in survival mode, 'like' never factored into it.

I have to relearn what I like. Addictions, alcohol and cigarettes apparently don't count.

Power | Fighting Back | Compassion

Dove

Power, I have never had it. I fear people with it. They use it to hurt, to force you to bend to their will, to take what they want. People with power have no morals, they don't have to, the legal system is a game for them. A way to stomp on the powerless, rub in the pain and humiliation and remind you how worthless you are. I learnt this the hard way.

I am terrified of men with power, my father, the judges, the coven, and later the predators who sensed my brokenness and vulnerability. All used it to hurt me, to satisfy themselves, to make money because they could.

They wielded power with relish, choosing who lives or dies. I soon learnt how powerless I was in life, no matter how hard I fought, I could never save myself or any of the other girls. I'd fight and fight to save them, worsening my fate and theirs, leaving blood on my hands, guilt, shame, and knowledge my abusers held all the power. I could never save them or myself. I was powerless over my own body; I had no control over what was done to it.

I was powerless to even save my own babies, I fought, screamed, nothing worked. Those with power beat me, held me down, aborted and dragged me away, vomiting and bleeding, to be hosed off. Just to make sure I knew who was boss.

The people I was hurt most by were the ones meant to use that power to protect me. My father gave me to them in return for career advancement and to fulfil sadistic desires. I was powerless, worthless. How could he do that to me? How revolting a child must I have been?

Now I box, I work out. A desperate, pathetic, useless attempt to feel strong, in control, have power over my body, who touches it and how. To never have to watch another girl being hurt. Until some asshole comes along and shatters the illusion.

Gabrielle

When the university put me in a mental institution
    the university had power. I was powerless.

When my parents used to belt me when I was young,
    my parents had the power. I was powerless.

When my brother sexually abused me when I was a child,
    he had the power. I was powerless.

Men have power.

They know if you like them.

So, they take up power.

They are emotionally decompartmentalized.

They take up power against you.

Male academics are strange creatures.

They have power.

Claire

Fighting back means look at his back and don't follow.
Fighting back means here is my hand, the palm of my hand,
see it, it is a stop sign. Fighting back means not lying down
and dying every time I am confronted, means asking what I feel,
what do I want, what do I need, fighting back.

Donna

Fighting back means a strength so fierce, so deep,
   so profound that dragons prowl on football grounds.

Lions surround me.

Angels beat drums.

Fighting back is like ecstasy.

Dionysian rhythms.

Safety chants.

Nikki

Fighting back means speaking out, being honest and holding up the truth. It's throwing the truth of our experience into the light, like a hook to the lie's jaw.

It's a fight where we speak our truths, and fight to never be silenced again. The fight is an act of love, to ourselves and each other.

Gabrielle

Compassion.

The best part of Graylands was the Aboriginal woman who after a patient said to her that she should call me her aunty, said "no she's my sister."

The last eight weeks

Lauren

The last eight weeks have taken me places I never thought I would go. Every assumption or expectation I have had on this journey has been shifted, challenged or played out in surprising ways. At first, I felt like I was a fraud. I downplayed my trauma and my suffering. I have learnt a lot about how I lived with this for so many years without telling a soul. Writing this, I feel a sense of peace. Birds are chatting outside and I'm pouring out my innermost thoughts and feelings alongside a group of women whom my admiration for cannot be put into words. I am thankful for them and everything they have taught me, and for everything they have shared, so often mirroring my own experience of living with this burden but travelling on their own unique and powerful paths. The past eight weeks have shown me how much I disconnect from my body. I feel like my relationship with my body has just been birthed. I still feel disconnected, but I'm on a trajectory now. All the bodily pain and suffering my life has been punctuated with has come into a new focus. From feeling unable to coordinate my movement well enough to play sport, to the hypervigilant and constant clamminess, chronic neck and back tension, severe abdominal pain, digestive issues, cancer. I don't see these things on a distinct plane anymore. They are interwoven with the anxiety and depression, the drinking and drugging, the mindless sex, the self-hatred. I feel stronger for feeling these connections. I feel further along the path. I feel proud of who I am and who I am becoming. *What I'm really trying to say is* I can feel myself shifting. It's slow and it's painstaking, at times terrifying. I still feel like I'm under attack. Like my own body wants me to feel pain, like my mind is lashing out because I deserve it. But I know what this is now. Knowing other survivors changes everything. It changes my perspective of my struggle and my perspective of *the* struggle.

Story is powerful. I feel so proud to have been part of this story. I'm glad it's not ending here. What I'm really trying to say is I have hope again. Hope that I can get better, that it's possible. That telling my story alongside the stories of this formidable group of women matters. I know it matters. So, I won't shut up anymore.

Donna

The last eight weeks have been a ride, smooth sailing.
Wind in hair. We held oars. We moved in rhythm. A storm hit.
We rode through it. No worse than what anyone has already
felt or seen. The last eight weeks I tried to be strong and then
I realised I wasn't trying. I was strong. I am strong.
We are strong.

The last eight weeks they spoke to me about my feelings,
my body, my disconnected body, my mind, my disconnected
mind, my shame, our shame, the secrets in our head. She told
on rape. She told on incest. She told on Church. She told
on father, on mother. I dreamt of brother. Last night, again.
He shouldn't have touched me.

Incest is the first breakthrough. As though this is something
to be proud of. The first marker. Then comes the dark images.
I'm waiting. I'm hearing. The screams. She told on neighbour.
They were all complicit. She told on them. The many.
She was outnumbered. She was powerless. I said, "you've all
got agency," deeply aware that wasn't true. Sometimes you are
a victim. I accepted my status and then I grew. I accepted my
status and got power. The last eight weeks were not meant to
be like this, but it was never meant to be like this. Let's face it.
It shouldn't have to be like this. It shouldn't have been.

The last eight weeks she smiled. She cried. She laughed.
She got angry. She could have beaten you so hard if given
a chance. She could have screamed so hard if given a chance.
Cold, cold, cold. Black and blue.

She could *have spit* in your face so hard. The rage was there,
and I welcomed it.

The last eight weeks she broke silence.

She told on you. And you. And you. She told you. And you.
And you. She told me. The last eight weeks she gave me
confidence. She told me, and me, and me, again, and again,
and again. And I wanted her to tell me again and again and
again, because I hid for so long and never knew what to say
or how to say it, anything, like my head and my thoughts got

so clammed up, clammy shells, I couldn't breathe, and I didn't know that was called trauma or dissociation or terror. I didn't know we were supposed to talk about it. Cos, they said don't you fucking talk about it. And we did. The last eight weeks, we talked about it. Told. Told. Told about it. What about it? Let her tell you about it. Come so close I want to listen while she tells you about it. The last eight weeks, she's gonna tell you all about it.

Gabrielle

I feel so blessed to have been in this writing group. I learnt how to punch, and I imagined the faces of my abusers as I punched the punching bag.

I wrote about how my abuse brought about other bad experiences in my life like *mental illness* and like being incarcerated in a mental institution. Of being seen as *the mad lady* at my university in Western Australia.

I was just seen as *the mad lady* and locked away because I was sexually abused as a child and an adult.

The workshop helped me realise I have experienced worse isolation than lockdown. I had been isolated in a mental institution. Whilst in lockdown I could still go outside. In the workshop I got to write about my body, about isolation and about power.

It was an honour to meet all the beautiful women in the group and to learn from their experiences, to understand why they felt negative because of their abuse.

Also, this week I got followed home by a man from the Ezymart.

I called the police. I felt uneasy with the idea of having sex with men. I thought I might identify as a lesbian instead of bi-sexual.

Julie

The last eight weeks have been a rollercoaster for me

I am here in my mind

But my body's not free

I just want the world to know

Just what it means

To regain my power

And fill my needs

I am so restricted in what I can do

But I am blessed with the writing

And I will see it through

The trauma has been

So intense in my life

It's hard to look forward

It's always a fight

Each time it happened

I thought something was wrong

Wrong with my actions, my body and thoughts

How could it happen so many times

I still carry the guilt

But I want to leave it all behind

The workshops have shown me

I really can grow

Inside my mind, my body and soul

So much was taken

From me all my life

I will never get those years back

But I will try and try

Friendships are hard

And they take so much trust

What do they want from me

To hurt me so much

Our bonds grow larger

And the trust starts to come in

Sharing our stories

From deep within

Each day is a challenge

And I never feel clean

I want to push down these walls

And let people in

I know it takes time

And I'm willing to share

All those horrible memories

That I really can't bear

Every day I search for one thing

That makes me feel stronger

Or puts power back within

I just want to cry

And let it all out

I need to release

But I'm not sure how

I'm out of my body

And just looking down

What I see is so much trauma

I want to scream and shout

Paranoia sets in

And makes it all worse

Always checking that my story gets heard

I see the people

They really are there

They scare me to death

Those bastards beware

Khale

The last eight weeks have taken me to some strange places. I have been carrying around these traumas for so long, hardly breathing them to anyone, and then suddenly, with much anxiety, I was in this group where it was OK to talk about them. No one asked what I was wearing or if I was drunk. No one tried to change the topic of conversation or make me be quiet. Everyone just held space for me week after week as I shared my feelings and memories of times past, shared what I have always considered to be my most shameful and disgusting secrets.

Listening to everyone's stories each week just felt like a new heartbreak. Sometimes I felt like the wind was knocked out of me, my vivid imagination picturing such evil acts being committed against these women who I knew only as strong and kind. I am always left floored at how truly evil some people can be, that they could do such cruel things to women and children.

It's been such a jarring experience each week to get so deeply entrenched in our collective trauma, to hear each other and cry for one another, then immediately exorcise the sadness from my body. It feels like as we share our secrets, I can feel the hook-like feet of depression trying to grapple onto me, trying to take hold. But before they get a chance to really dig in, I'm up, I'm moving, I'm too fast, you can't catch me, I'll run, I'll punch, there's no way you can get your hooks into me.

It feels like the sadness keeps trying to stick to me, but because I won't stop moving it can never take hold.

By the time we've completed the hour of boxing I'm exhausted, but the sadness, the trauma, feels so much farther away than it did at the start. I still remember everything, it's still deeply saddening, but it doesn't feel like it's inside me anymore, like a rock in my guts. It feels like things I know, things I can talk about, but it's a narrative that I can control rather than the other way around. I feel more like my body is something useful, something that serves me, protects me, rather than something that just makes me a target for abuse.

I feel less angry at my body for being female, and more thankful to it for being capable.

Dove

The last eight weeks have held many challenges. We have literally seen the whole world and life as we know it turned on its head because of a virus.

I have learnt a lot about myself, faced fears and overcome challenges. I have faced my fear of cameras, even filmed video diaries and reached a point of *ok-ness* with them (the zoom version anyway). I'm proud of this as I never thought I would be able to do it. Overcoming fears are a powerful step forward.

I have stuck it out and shared an amazing eight weeks with eight other inspirational women. I have learnt I am not alone and that the pain, fears, and negative feelings I experience are normal for child sexual abuse survivors. The everyday struggles are normal, I am not a stupid, weak, useless freak.

I am learning I am stronger than I realize and that one day I may have something worthwhile to offer other survivors. That I may be able to help and give them hope.

I have allowed myself to be open and share things I would normally hide. Vulnerabilities, deep feelings, struggles and insecurities I normally keep to myself.

I have boxed and worked out, something that has helped me survive and stay sane. I have loved sharing it with other survivors, sharing the feelings of empowerment and the release of hurt and anger.

Nikki

The last eight weeks have been a physical and emotional journey. It's been a process of feeling, and discovery and working through both. I feel a sense of connection — connection to myself, to my centre, to my story, to my writing, my body and an incredible group of women who are inspiring and inspire.

I feel like I've drawn strength from this group and am so grateful for the process and its timing. This pandemic has been like a time of forced reflection — and what better time to confront one's inner demons than in a slow-motion apocalypse?

What I really want to say is thank you. Thank you for giving me tools and time to tell my story and expressing my feelings about what's occurred. Thank you for never making me feel like my story was too much, or that I was not enough. Thank you for reaffirming that.

What I really want to say is we are all so strong — I draw inspiration from this group in dark moments, and your words stay with me like lights in the dark.

What I really want to say is I'm looking forward with a sense of calm I didn't have even six weeks ago. I look forward because I'm acknowledging a past, I shut away, and moving through its repercussions. I don't think I'll ever be over it or free of it — but it's starting to feel less.

I named him — and the world didn't collapse, he didn't get me from the grave. Maybe I'm starting to realise he can't hurt me anymore — he can't hurt anyone anymore.

The last eight weeks have given me gifts — this group, a voice, and a sense of connection — I am so grateful for that.

What I really want to say is the sun is warming me and I feel a sense of peace in this moment that is so rare and beautiful I could cry. Even as my hand aches from writing and we are spread across a city I feel connected to you all, and to myself. This is a beautiful moment.

And now in a classic turn I feel a little awkward and almost ashamed to have been so raw and honest — I know sometimes my positivity is too much. But fuck it — it's how I feel. Fucken love you powerful queens — stay strong, stay badass, stay kind. You are heroes in my eyes.

ROUND
TWO

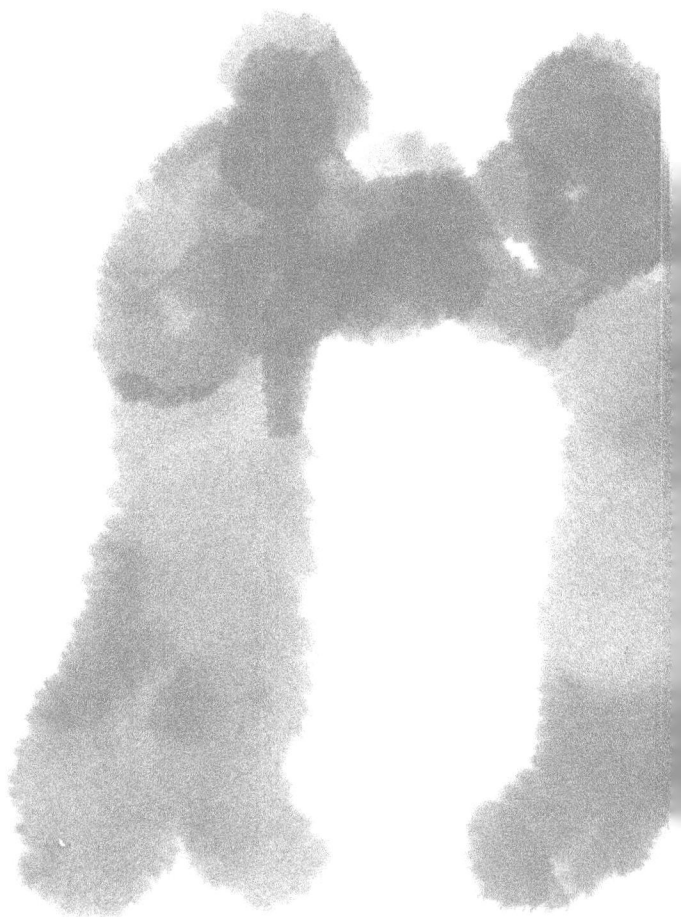

About Round Two

Donna

By Round Two, I was clear on how boxing is a mode of practice that can aid survivors' mental health and wellbeing. I wanted to deepen this exploration and more consciously explore the interplay between the physical and mental.

Like most survivors, I have struggled with control, being controlling, or being controlled, and I found relaxing and being present very difficult to sustain. During training, maintaining control and precision is juxtaposed with movement, rhythm, flow, and agility. Boxing is a form of mindfulness; the expressiveness of the movements enables one to safely practice holding both tension and release.

The prompts picked in this round concentrated on the important principles of boxing, being grounded, focused, fluid, powerful and vulnerable. The prompts evolved as a response to these ideas, continuing to gently encourage the survivor to get in touch with their underlying thoughts and beliefs surrounding their trauma. Examples of prompts are, writing a love letter to a part of the body, talking to the nervous system, and writing about what *trusting the process* means. By bringing this thinking and feeling into awareness, we then moved into a boxing drill. Any feelings that arose could be channelled into a new mode, moving from mind into outer expression, through body.

Round Two Writing Prompts

I am back here because | I begin again | Today

Being a survivor | Denial

Trusting the process | Being on guard | Relaxation

When I listen | I listened
Two feet on the ground | Being present

Write a conversation between you
and your nervous system
Write a love letter to a part of your body
Write all the things you hate and all the things you love

Reclaiming me | Self-esteem

He / she / they / I pushed... | I turned...

I thought I was going to
It's hard to speak out because | What it takes

Intimacy | Effects of my abuse
Write a love letter to your inner child
What is meaningful?

Trauma

Silence

Writing + Boxing =

Choose one prompt at a time from each grouping above.
Turn your timer on for 10 minutes and write non-stop using
the prompt as your starter line.

I am back here because | I begin again Today

Donna

I am back here because I need to bandage my soul.

I need to listen to the women share and tell their stories
to help me tell mine.

I need to find out who I was before it all happened.

And when I say *it*, I don't even know what *it* is.

I just know that my childhood is black and filled with feelings
of darkness and terror and underneath my skin, I feel dirt
and disgust still that I can't pin on a clear narrative, so I think
if I am forced to write, not forced, encouraged, I must write,
then maybe it will come out — its cryptic.

I am back here because I said I would be.

It gives me purpose.

I like writing.

I love boxing.

I like listening to the women.

I want to be heard.

I want to break free of said clichés.

Of feeling bad.

Just change it. *Think differently*.

I do. It's buried deep. It's only there in the quiet.

Mainly at night, in bed, when I *check in*, I feel the discomfort;
the pain climbs through me, the little terrified voices.
The messy, messy blackness. The hushing. The rollercoaster
maze. That's why I read, so my eyes get droopy, and I fall
asleep. Left alone, with my thinking, my partner breathing
quietly. I live in too much black. When I move, I break free.

I am back here because this is a practice, that I trust, that makes sense, that seems to work, that seems to move something or form something.

Connection on page.

Connection in body.

Connection in mind.

Connection with them.

I am back here because of the abuse. Because of silencing.

Because of them. Because of needing to do something all the fucking time, because it is pressing, because if I don't, I might die, sometimes that doesn't matter, but I don't want to let them win. I am back here because of light shining greater than darkness. Light. Because of healing wounds.

Khale

I am back here because my trauma is still so big, so present in my life. I still have PTSD (post traumatic syndrome). A psychologist once told me that you don't ever really recover from complex PTSD. I really, really hope that she's wrong. I try to be optimistic and imagine there will be a time in my life when I won't have vivid flashbacks that take days to recover from. That there will be a time when I won't have to be woken from nightmares by my wife and just held for half the night because I'm afraid to go back to sleep.

I'm back here because I don't know exactly what I need to heal, but I know this is helping. I didn't understand how much I needed this until I was right in it. I didn't know how important it was to be listened to without being told to talk about more pleasant things or to not talk about it if it makes you so upset. I didn't know I had been seeking validation and understanding for so long.

There is such an immense relief that comes from being able to share my shame and not be judged for it. To let my dark and dirty secrets see the light of day and breathe, so that just for ten minutes they aren't rotting inside me, growing, and festering and getting ready for the next time they will spring into mind unannounced and shut my whole life down for an hour or a day or a week. When other peoples' ears are on my shame, people who I know aren't judging me, then for just a few minutes I start to feel like maybe it's not my fault that these things happened, because it's none of our faults that we are here. I start to look upon myself with some of the compassion I have for the others who are here. It is such an immense relief to be talking about these secrets yet not be hating myself for them for just a few minutes. It feels like being inside out, but in a good way. Like the light can touch all those parts of me that have been hidden.

Julie

I begin again down a road of uncertainty

Holding and watching what lies ahead of me

Each day is different

It's never the same

One day my words won't be in vain

And hope that I'm free

I want the world to see the real me

I begin again and each time is so different

Finding my voice

Lets me begin again

I don't want to repeat what I've already done

I want to start afresh

And let my emotions run wild

I find each week my voice for a while

I want to be open

And not shy away

Hoping my story

Will help someone else one day

I begin again with the boxing as well

Hoping that real soon

I can punch and scream

Whatever happens I'll show the real me

I am so self-conscious

And sometimes withdrawn

But I feel with this group

I am safe right from dawn

I want to learn

And use what I have

Always searching for something

From up above
I pray really hard
To someone, I know
Looking for answers
To help me get through
I begin this journey
With one thought in sight
To follow my heart
And follow the light

Lauren

I begin again every time it visits me, and I lose myself and I fall in a heap and crawl back up to find air. It could be a small thing. A phrase, an off-handed comment. A challenge that goes wrong. An obstacle. A splinter. A leaky hole that opens in the structure I have made for myself to move around in. I slip and lose my footing. Doubt creeps in. Do I even have a right to be here? Who am I in this structure? Where am I? Can I trust it? I'm not safe. Maybe I'm safe? I'm not sure if I'm safe. I'll go for a run. I'll stop doing all the bad things. I'll do self-care. Assemble the ingredients to take myself back, to find my foundation. I slip again. I must have fucked up. I didn't act it out right. I didn't patch the right hole. Another hole has appeared in a place I wasn't expecting. I begin again. Will I do things differently this time? I've learned things. New rules, new practices. Will they work this time? I don't know if I can trust them. There are no guarantees. I'm back in the place where I'm waiting for bad things to happen, where badness is built into my existence. I hit rock bottom. There's no way out. I want it to end. I don't know what to do. I don't know what is real. I don't know where the exits are. I am scared. I feel trapped. I take stock. I zone out. I do the things I have done many times before, while all my bones scream opposition, sneer at me that there's no point, that it won't help. But I know this is a place I am visiting. Even though it feels like I will never leave, that I can't escape. I do it anyway, fighting every urge to self-destruct. I keep going and hope that in time it will pass, that I will feel better.

Nikki

I feel the trap closing, unable to get out. How is it that a socially constructed net makes me feel more trapped and restrained than chains and ties ever could? How is it that this feeling of being manipulated and gaslighted has me shaking, crying, silent and screaming, frozen in terror?

As the fear takes over, I lose time to moments long passed.

I awake shaking and shaken — I come back to myself as an adult, while the child within cowers and cries.

I lie there staring at the floor and holding the child in a way not possible then.

I exhale — acknowledge that the memories won this round and get up off the floor. Round Two. I begin again.

I remind myself that I am no longer a child, and I have the power to leave now. I will protect her.

I will continue to show up, continue to do the work and be accountable to myself. I have, and I will continue. A step back doesn't undo my journey. It doesn't minimise my progress, my worth or strength. This moment of vulnerability is strength. I will keep walking forward and kicking in the blockades. Sometimes I will fall, sometimes I will stop for a time. But every time I will gather myself and move forward. Even if it's a fucking crawl — I will move the earth round.

Each time I will remain and outlast them. Even if I'm knocked off this mountain, back to base, or even below. I will get up, dust off and climb again. You won't beat me old man.

I begin again.

Claire

Today I wake up to myself today I make up to myself today I wake up in the room I have put together today I wake up needing to pee but can't move today I wake up to needing to move today I wake up needing to move out of what I have slept in today my sheets are white and almost clean today I don't remember going to sleep today I realise I woke in freeze to live or die if I play dead they will not kill me today I woke up needing to pee not being able to get out of bed to getting out of bed what selves to gather around me to bring together to put feet on the ground stand under water under the whys of where today I got in the shower cover my face and lower back today I woke up got out of bed and had a shower the only escape is to break routine this soap of sell usually go out into the garden I met the page I meet my feelings on the page I am not protecting others I am sad and angry pulling weeds we don't pull weeds because we think they will never grow back again I pull weeds so that what I have planted can grow the clover that does not belong here has grown through the salt bush I have planted here that is indigenous the less robust plants have not survived me not weeding I have hot lemon the water the lemon tree I have had for years has lemons on it I asked my lover to pee on it the lemon tree has lemons on it I need to get out of the house off the page I go shopping to get out of the self around this house this house that I work and sleep in I remember the police commissioner saying on T.V. don't fight back you might get hurt my boyfriend and society demanding the details it's only rape if you have bruises all over you and me feeling guilty I didn't I froze if I play dead this sweat dripping in my face his sweat dripping in my face when there is no exit I exit myself

Dove

Today. Relief it's not yesterday or any of the ones before that.
The end of the week. A week that has changed everything.

Disclosure, today the dust settles, my mind grapples to
comprehend what I now know. A new unknown, new fear,
I gave the knife back, maybe I should have kept it. I didn't
know what I know today.

I failed, suffered not enough. The blackness, it spread far further
than I ever imagined, insidious, lethal, I saved no-one.

Today my heart breaks, I am full of rage, fear, brokenness,
and shame. I failed. Fool! I thought I could contain it if
I suffered enough.

I struggle to remember who I am; it can change so quickly.
Today as the dust settles, I once again face my fear of cameras,
of sharing, which has grown exponentially since last time.
I prepare to expose myself again. All that I want to hide.

I feel raw, all that I wanted to hide has been dragged out of me,
what I feared most is fact. Ugliness seeps from every exposed
pore for all to see.

Today, I at least have a safe space to share, nothing will be
forced from me, dragged out. My weapons won't be taken away,
brokenness and vulnerability are ok.

Being a Survivor | Denial

Lauren

Being a survivor really sucks sometimes. I am frequently brought back to the realisation that survival is never done. It is a constant striving for agency, safety, justice, joy. It is hard. But I am strong. I am proud. I can be vulnerable and hold my space. I can be honest and demand respect. I hold these juxtapositions in my survivor heart.

Dove

Being a survivor is shit. It's a long dark tunnel. It is clawing your way out of a deep, cold well, only to be knocked back down over and over when you finally glimpse light. Each time thinking the well could not possibly get deeper. It is lonely, isolating, discouraging, exhausting.

Donna

Being a survivor is a stupid thing.

It's cancer victims or war victims or surviving volcano eruptions.

Being a survivor means surviving through a horrible trauma or traumas where it shatters body, mind and soul and it's like wearing a badge for participating. Like, it's good you showed up, but what does it really matter? You didn't win.

Julie

Being a survivor

A word I've just learnt

What does it mean

I just want to blurt

It's only been said

A few times to me

And slowly I'm learning

A SURVIVOR

That's me

How does it feel

To shout it out loud

I want to be free

And also be found

Being a survivor

It slowly sinks in

Right in my heart

Khale

Being a survivor is fucked. It means always being a victim, having people look at you with pity. Just having people look at you at all is terrifying. Do they know? Can they tell? Does everyone see me as broken, damaged goods? *Survivor* is a strong word, but I don't feel strong. I feel like garbage left in the rain that no one wants to clean up. Smelly and soggy and just getting walked on until it is part of the concrete.

Julie

Denial....so many people in my life live by this word

It's got them through

Not knowing what to do

But my heart breaks into small pieces

Not being heard

I put up my defences

Will they ever know

How much it hurts me

To not be validated

Or hugged

Or nurtured

Claire

Denial is beautiful. It is a walk in the park with deciduous trees
in autumn. Its compartments of a fold-out suitcase, don't unzip
that compartment. Denial is survival. Denial is exhausting,
holding up the mask over my face that weighs like gold.
Golden leaves rush, rust gold falls from trees. Denial is a smile,
hidden behind that Luna Park gaping smile.

Khale

I am probably in denial of a lot of things. Maybe I'm an addict.
Maybe I'm an alcoholic. I don't know. What I'm really trying
to say is, I worry about myself. What will it be that kills me
if not myself? Can I survive my mind long enough to develop
cancer, liver disease, renal failure? I'm daily denying that
I completely fucked my body up with years of starvation.

Dove

Denial is dangerous. It should be bliss, but it leaves you open,
vulnerable. Denial is footsteps outside the bedroom door
that signal danger, the rattling door is wind, that men ever
care about you as a person, that your friends' partner is safe.

Lauren

Denial is pretending a problem doesn't exist. Denial is harm.
Denial is mere translation. The pain moves to my abdomen,
shoulders, neck, digestive system. My body remembers
and bears witness.

Trusting the process | Being on Guard Relaxation

Julie

Trusting the process

And breaking down the fortress

So many barriers

Where will it all carry us

Into the unknown

I place my trust in my own hands

Hoping that one day I will make a stand

My mind is full of conflict and hate

I'll go full steam ahead

And break down those layers

The abuse that I faced

Will never leave me

Horror and torment I live in my dreams

Only when I wake

There's nothing in between

I see their faces

And I'll never forget

All that prodding and poking

In places I regret

Why didn't people notice

I was living in a bubble

I didn't want to talk

I didn't want any trouble

They said I daydreamed

But now I really know

DISASSOCIATION is a word that flows

I have lost so much time

And my childhood is endless

It's only now that I trust this whole process

In so many directions

My heart has been torn

Broken in pieces

I'll fight for a new dawn

Sifting through the baggage

Wondering if I have enough luggage

To process my thoughts

With the tools I hold close

I am in charge now

Of my mind and my body

I won't let anyone abuse me

Or take advantage of me

I'm scared of my past

But it doesn't define

The person I am inside

Dove

Trusting the process is hard. I'm sick of the fucking process, it never ends, a sick joke, but I guess that's not the process's fault.

I want to heap blame for the pain I feel on the process, but that isn't right either. It is not the fault of the process that it is so bloody long!

If it weren't for the process, I would be back at the beginning. Would I be better off? I know I would be dead.

At first, I embraced it, believing I could get through it. I had no idea it would be so long or what was waiting for me.

I now know what was wrong with me. It's my life, I wanted to know what had happened to me, not realizing just how much or how evil it was. The process went on, each new memory an escalation. Surely it can't get worse, surely there can't be more, I gave up saying that years ago.

The process now terrifies me, but I have no choice but to continue. It's there, all the pain and memories and they will come whether I like it or not.

Now I wait to see what the process will bring this time. I am scared, I don't want to know. I am being prostituted again, in a seedy, low light building. At least I am 15 this time. I can hear what's happening, I know multiple perpetrators await me, maybe a camera. I know they are sick and twisted, I know this will not be my only job for the evening and I know what I will find through the door will be really, really, bad. I know death and blood are involved. I wish I could stay out of there, but I can't, the parts need to be heard. So, the process continues, I will walk through the door and see, feel and hear what awaited me. I will shake, feel sick, ache, cry, and box my way through.

The process owns me now, there is no escape. I am stronger for it, yet completely broken. My family is broken, my relationships, all because of me.

I don't want to do it anymore. I've had enough. I hate the process. I don't want to go through that door.

Khale

I have been on guard for SO long. I was hypervigilant even as a young person, even before I could remember anything. The first time I ever rode in a car with boys, hiding in the backseat, terrified, becoming more and more panicked even though these were FRIENDS that I hung out with regularly. They were supposed to drive me home but finally I couldn't take it anymore and shouted "I live here! Let me out!" on the side of the highway. I walked the last 40 minutes home in the dark at midnight because that felt less scary than sitting in the backseat next to a boy for a moment longer.

The problem is, even when you are hypervigilant, even when you do everything *right*, you still aren't safe. That night in St Kilda, it was 2am and I had only been hanging out with girls all night. "My place is close; you should crash rather than going home so late". It seemed safe. SHE seemed safe. She was a friend. She offered me a drink and I just accepted it gratefully and went to bed. She had been so kind to me all night. But she changed, so suddenly and so completely. She was holding me down, forcing my legs apart, yelling at me, pushing me, demanding I submit. She was so strong and I was so small. Her weight felt like so much, she was so angry, I kept trying to force my legs together and pull away but she held my wrists so tight.

The next day she apologised. She said, "Last night, that wasn't me, I'm not like that." I just wanted to go home. When I got home I undressed for a shower to wash the night off me. I was so shocked to see myself in the mirror and see all the bruises. My arms, my thighs, my stomach. It looked brutal. In a way it was perfect, because for once I looked exactly on the outside how I felt on the inside. Ruined. Raped. Broken. Ugly. Something that needs to be thrown away.

Sometimes I just don't know how to navigate the world when you can NEVER be safe. Am I an idiot for still wanting to trust people, to hope that there are people in this world who truly would never hurt you? Even my ex-girlfriends all got violent with time.

This is the first time I've been in a relationship where I can honestly say everything is always consensual. It took me a long time to believe that maybe this time, things are different. For years I kept expecting that one day, she too would get angry, would be forceful, would start pushing. But she never did.

Lauren

Being on guard. What am I guarding? *What I'm really trying to say is* I'm so used to being let down. Being unseen, unheard. Too sensitive, too passionate, too much. The one who can't *let things go*. My experience as a person who suffers from mental illness and trauma is one where I am constantly *gaslighted*. People don't want to hear it. I remember feeling angry and cynical at a work fundraiser for mental health. People like to think they would offer meaningful support to someone with mental health issues, but when it enters their periphery and demands their attention and time, when the sufferer doesn't act the way they think they should act, people don't bother in my experience. The stigma is still so real. It costs careers, friendships, lives. It's complete bullshit. It's tiring. I'm tired. I'm tired of not being able to move through the world freely. That I can't mobilise my support system for depression the way I can for cancer. That I still have to be careful who I share my experience with because they will start to equate my mental illness with my personality. If mental illness demands anything from anyone, they will insidiously *gaslight* you with deflection, deferral, inaction, so that they don't have to feel bad about being callous and unsupportive. I am so exhausted. If we all could just be honest and show some compassion, and actually listen, these things might start to change. I'm tired of being an advocate. I stand up for myself, push myself to the brink, almost let it kill me. I still haven't worked out how to do it sustainably. Not doing it would kill me faster. What a choice to make. A choice many people won't acknowledge exists. I'm so fucking angry and tired and this is certainly not going to be my most articulate piece of writing. But through writing, recording, sharing my story, I reclaim it. Again, and again. It boosts my energy. Maybe one day people might read my story and understand. Is that naïve? I've been told I expect too much from people, like being treated with the dignity and respect that I deserve. Often, I think the only reason this is so hard for me is because the people who don't live life with trauma tune out. They don't care. Injustice that doesn't affect them isn't injustice at all. I need to *let it go*.

Claire

Relaxing is taking the chain I hang over my shoulders off. It drags along the ground as I walk. To take it off I have to get my hands underneath it. It is incredibly heavy. I have to be Hercules. But I get my hands under it and lift it enough just to slip from underneath it. Then what? I'm so fucken light I think my head is going to leave my body. No, that is something else. I feel like my head is going to detach from my body when I am pinned down and asked to stay with the truth. Too much fucken truth, truth like treacle, the syrup dumplings my mother made sticking to the pan, as cloying as betrayal, sickly sweet as amber, the insect in the amber before it is amber. Sap I can't get off my fingers and being bitten by bull ants. It's super-hot, I smell bursting eucalypt pods. It is in FNQ (Far North Queensland), there are ant hills. A walk in the bush outside, it is safer than inside. Looking at myself for three hours, it's like a mirror meditation, it's dangerous. I see how strained I am, can't hide it anymore in the veil of youth.

I go cold at betrayal, I invite betrayal. Betrayal is going cold. The inside of an empty removal truck, the dripping tap into a metal sink. Relaxing is escape, relaxation CD. Go somewhere else, connect to higher self. Relaxing is being present, is feeling my heart stir. Relaxing is feeling safe, unclench, stop holding my left shoulder up bracing for the next hit. Relaxing is believing the floor won't drop me but it has before or I have dropped to the floor or the floor has dropped away and I'm pinned to the walls with centrifugal force. Fall. Relaxation is hope, grasping onto twigs that break, can't get a foothold to pull myself out of this. Relaxation is a lie to myself. If I relax truly I'm vulnerable to the memories. If I keep pretending I build a new me, like a Lego person, there are not many choices of pieces, it is very generic. Relaxation is the meditator's reality. I rebuild *a me* with scarves and mirrors. I construct a being word after word. I form a sentence, a walking sentence. I can get up and walk, put one foot to the floor then the next, put one word down then the next. Words are drips of water filled with light hanging off leaves, that tension holding onto the tip. Relaxation is letting go.

When I listen | I listened
Two feet on the ground | Being present

Lauren

When I listen I can tune into the memory. Not in my thoughts but my skin, my fingers, my throat, my legs, my feet. If I keep listening it is there in my abdomen. It visits whenever I struggle or feel strain, stress, or if I don't feel safe. When I listen I'm forced to acknowledge the weight of this impact, its ongoing nature, its weaving in my bones, in the physical pathways of my brain. When I listen I am reminded of scale, of my lizard brain, of my competing faculties. I am reminded that the work will take time. When I listen I can sense my ability to grow, to learn, to shift, but it mostly feels different to what I expect, as I unlearn the capitalist mantras of wellness and healing, of massages and flotation tanks that lead to peace and salvation. Of the empty promises of empowerment. I am reminded of grace, and grit. When I listen I see a path of pain laid out in front of me, but also behind me. I see the resilience and hope and love at the heart of my drive for survival. When I listen I feel the reality of my existence as a whole system, my brain and my body the result of thousands of years of evolution and conditioning, reckoning with and adapting to this new domesticated sphere. A place where we understand ourselves in sections. We deal with our issues with extreme specificity and avoid looking at ourselves as whole. When I listen I can sense this whole. I feel closer to the ground, more real, more alive. I can feel the plasticity of my brain and the responses of my organs. I can see the ramifications of injustice as shame through a cross-section of our society. When I listen I see the reality of my abuser, not as a monster but a broken and sick boy, whose behaviour is reinforced by a system that serves the powerful.

Julie

When I listen
I hear a faint breath
Waiting for the moment
That his time will end
I am not afraid
As I hold his hand
I feel comfort all around me
I weep quietly in the stands
I sing him some songs
And I hope he can hear
The breathing gets weaker
And morning appears
The blind is down
And the wind blows in
All through the night
I am talking to him
The nurses around me
Give me comfort and light
Please God take him
Sometime in the night
I hear the phone ring
But no change is upon me
I say a quiet prayer
And just wait patiently

When I listen

No words are spoken

The warmth of his hand

He lies peacefully like the sand

Only a wave

As his chest rises and falls

And then it happened

Please don't let me fall

Two short breaths

And he was gone

He looked like an angel

Don't be forlorn

I say goodbye

To my beautiful dad

To be forever with him

I feel so sad

Donna

When I listen, I hear voices inside of me, split off from me. They hurt. They are sad.

They feel disgusting and bad and ashamed. When I listen, I ignore, because it is draining to hear how sad and bad and dirty I am.

Sometimes, when I listen, I soothe, I comfort and try to be kind, as though I was dealing with a small child who was coming to me hurt and terrified.

When I listen, I want to break down and cry and heave, but my pride protects me. I keep working.

I listened and I loved and then I dreamt I was on a boat with hundreds of students, and it started to sink and turn upwards, plunging into the depths of water.

Later, I was standing outside the boat, which had turned into a gigantic fish, like Jonah. Everyone was inside and I had to slice open the fish to save them.

When I listen, I am afraid. I cannot listen for long. I dissociate. My mind switches to a different neural pathway. I am easily distracted. When I listen to my breath at night, and I listen to the pain in my body, I sense images of horror and all that is trapped inside me screams to come out.

When I listen, I hear wailing.

When I listen, I go blank.

When I listen, I cannot hear.

When I listen, I hear birds and heavy breathing and terror gripping my body.

When I listen, I pray to die and feel guilty of my existence.

When I listen, I tune out to hear vague sounds on the radio.

When I listen, I wonder if and when it will ever be calm and safe and gentle and sweet and safe and calm and gentle and sweet and safe and gentle and sweet and safe and calm and gentle and sweet. When I listen, I am interrupted.

Khale

When I listened, everything scared me. It should have been such an easy thing. We're going to a party, it's all people I don't know, but they're my girlfriend's friends, she knows them, she knows they are safe. There are men here, but I just ignore them. I stay in small groups of women. But the night gets long and no one leaves. We are staying the night here. Shouldn't people be leaving? It's late. I want to go to bed. The host shows me our room. My girlfriend checks that I am OK then re-joins the party. From in that room, all I can hear are the men. Why are they so loud? They laugh, push each other, challenge each other. I know what happens when men drink and become brave. Why are they all still here? What if one of them comes in here? I check for a lock, but the door doesn't have one. There's not even any furniture I can push against the door. How can I stay safe here? I'm sure one of them will stumble in here at any moment. I lay curled in a tiny ball in the corner, shaking, crying, forcing myself not to black out. Why does their obnoxious laughter make me feel so afraid? It feels like hours of being trapped in that terrified state before my girlfriend comes in to check on me again. She immediately comes to my aid, but sighs deeply. She resents these panic attacks so much. Always bringing her down, taking her away from the party. Now she has to sit here with her pathetic shaking little girlfriend when she wants to be drinking and laughing out there. I'm so sick of being a burden. I'm so sick of having to be looked after. I want to be able to sort myself out, but I can't do that until I can get somewhere SAFE.

I wish everywhere didn't feel unsafe to me. I'm sorry, I'm sorry, I always ruin your night. I'm sorry, I know you're sick of comforting me. I'm sorry, I know you wish I could just get over it. I do too. But these fears are buried so deep within me that I don't think I can get them out.

Dove

I listened and internalized everything they told me,
as young children do.

I listened when they said I was evil, wicked, naughty,
and needed to be punished.

I listened when they said I was dirty, disgusting, and shameful,
that my mum would leave if she knew how revolting I was,
that my brothers and I would be left with my dad.

I listened when they told me it was my purpose to please men,
that the mess meant I had pleased them, and God would be
happy with me.

I listened when they said I was disgusting and dirty
when the mess ran out of my body.

I listened when they said I was evil, disappointing
and a piece of shit when I rebelled or resisted.

Later, I listened when they said it was too late, I belonged
to them, a bride of Satan, the mark of the beast etched
on my ribs.

I listened when they said I had to pay my way with my body,
it is all I am good for.

I listened when they said I was one of the lucky ones
not to be marked, my throat still intact.

I listened when they said it was my fault, I was pregnant,
that I was a slut, that they once again had to fix my problem.

I listened when they said it was my fault, she was dead,
I had forced them to do it.

I listened when they said it was my fault the baby was dead,
that it was mine and I caused its death.

I listened when they said I can never escape, they owned me,
Satan was watching me.

Then came a point when I stopped listening, I heard,
I had no choice, but I didn't listen. I knew they would
do whatever they wanted regardless of what I did.

Nikki

Two feet on the ground, barefoot toes wiggling amongst
the dirt. I take root, dig deep, and remember — breathe in,
breathe out, observe.

The leaves above, swaying gently calms — breathe in,
breathe out in time with the sway. Come back to myself
and centre — literally grounded.

Know where I end and the world begins, connect, and go
deeper. Centre and breathe. I may not have a god, but I feel this
connection, one with nature that breathes in time with the sway.

The branches shade from the harsh, unforgiving light that
nurtures but burns deep. And stay marked and painful —
a memory that keeps on hurting.

The roots, the toes connecting and burrowing — connect back
to the centre and breathe. Bend and sway as a storm rages on —
remaining centred and grounded — it will pass, and sanctuary
will return.

What I really want to say is that the earth has nurtured
me in moments where nothing felt real — in those moments
it felt like only my feet could connect to the present and provide
calm. In moments of panic, of overwhelming emotions watching
the branches is one of the few things that helped. Two feet
on the ground, I breathe deep and centre. Open my eyes
and start forward.

What I really want to say is nature offers a silent wisdom
and connection back, a way forward. She endures,
overcomes, is burned, recovers. She is wise and calm,
yet strong and vicious. She is strength.

Two roots in the ground and arms raised up — she wears
her crown of leaves and endures beyond mortal years.

Claire

Being present.

This is a big one. I watch the person beside me like they are from another planet. Being present. I know, breathe. Being present is about feeling real. What is present. I know, breathe right now, I write. Sensory detail. Being aware of what is outside of me. Not just being inside my head, where what is inside my head is a great gelatinous blob that fills all space. Being present is looking at the house and saying I put this together. Do I recognize it? Looking at the plants in my house. Did I plant these? I was given this rug my feet are on by a rug seller who was kind and generous and wanted to repay us for giving him a free couch. The spiky balls from the Pilates teacher. Being present. In the present means not being in the past, fucken simple concept taken a lifetime to grasp. Being present, I don't achieve being present by being cut off from the past. The past made the present. The quilt on my couch was made in the past by my mother. She was halfway through it when she had a car accident that disabled one of her grandchildren, broke all her ribs, thought she would never finish it but she did. What we make, piece together, piece by piece is the present continuity. When there is no continuity there is no present. The present is between the past and the future. It's the life-force the waves of life force, the continuance. The present. Being present, there are things around me not just inside me, all is inside, everything is inside.

Dove

Being present is uncomfortable, it is facing reality,
it is fraught with danger.

It is acknowledging my weaknesses, feeling vulnerable
and sitting with it even though I don't want to.

It is not allowing myself to hide in a cloud of dissociation,
facing fears, and uncomfortable feelings of shame, disgust,
weakness, and pain.

It is acknowledging all the pain my body feels, all the damage
and problems instead of dissociating from and ignoring it.

It is to be afraid and aware of all the dangers of the world
and how powerless I am. It is to realize how little control
I really have.

Being present means facing up to all the things I don't want
to face. It's overwhelming, the scale of what happened
overwhelms and crushes me.

It is facing all the fears and awful feelings in a present
I do not want

Being present is drastically overrated.

Donna

Being present used to be an impossible task.

Led me to alcoholism.

Led me to panic attacks.

Led me to shaking. Regression.

Led me to dissociation.

Being present is unpleasant.

Night-time terrors.

Sometimes it is fun. Sensual.

Then I switch. Being present is momentary.

Being present is confusing.

Set me off.

Send me sideways.

Being present is not knowing.

I am present. Presenting. It is presenting a self who needs to operate in a moment. It is being able to perform with ease. It is not watching myself at a distance slightly to the left, seeing hands on paper. Objectively seeing body as object — pen in hand, that is not present — it is presenting me to myself — it is my form of present — it is self-conscious.

Being present; leads to body memories, bad dreams. I avoid it when I can. Being present is listening to the icky, irky, yukky, crawling over my skin. It is feeling electric current, snapshots of synapses, fizzing, momentary bouts of pain. Before a blanket of present denial goes up, covers the day.

Being present is new age hype, designed for the wealthy. It is a reality of fear, horror, pain, depression, guilt, and shame for the survivor. Being present is feeling. It sends me blank.

what I really want to say is, *what I really want to say is*,
what I really want to say is, *what I really want to say is*,
what I really want to say is, *what I really want to say is*,
what I really want to say is, *what I really want to say is*,
what I really want to say is, *what I really want to say is*,
what I really want to say is, *what I really want to say is…*

Khale

I feel like there is so much media and conversation about being present. *Mindfulness* they call it. My first introduction to mindfulness came from my dietitian teaching me how to eat. "You have to be present. Honour the meal. Think about what every bite means to your body." I couldn't think of anything worse. Eating was something I was forced to do, and I tried my hardest to distract myself as I choked down every meal. For years eating made me cry.

Being present means being alone with my thoughts. How terrifying. Every time I go for a long drive I end up in tears because spending too long in my own company is guaranteed to take me on a journey of all my worst memories and biggest mistakes.

I want to think of myself as an independent person, but the truth is, it's dangerous for me to spend too much time by myself. I get so sad, I get so dark, I get suicidal.

Be present. Observe your surroundings. Listen. Be aware of your thoughts. What can you feel? Smell? Hear? Taste? See? My mind learned to completely black out from a young age so that I wouldn't have to be present. I was spared from the worst of it by my dissociation. It seems like a betrayal to try to destroy that protective mechanism.

Why would I want to be present, to sit with my awful memories and wretched feelings? Why would I want to be with myself, the person I hate? Isn't it so, so much better to be distracted? To be doing and thinking literally anything else? Why is it so important to be present, to be mindful? Isn't it enough to just be functional?

Write a conversation between you and your nervous system | Write a love letter to a part of your body | Write all the things you hate and all the things you love

Lauren

Hey nervous system. It's me. Won't you let me go? I can't imagine a life where I am not trapped by you. Where I don't feel you guard the entrances to my body and soul, responding to everything as a threat. I don't know how you manage to work so hard. In a sense I feel sorry for you, that you feel so much responsibility for cutting me off from life. Keeping me away from danger. Sometimes, funnily, keeping me away from danger takes me to it. My own body becomes dangerous. I feel unsafe in my own skin. What kind of system is this? Not one that I'm happy with. Perhaps I would even protest against it. Why do you make me feel this way? Why does every interaction have a layer of anxiety, stress, uncertainty? Why must I work so hard just to move around in this world? Sometimes you make me question what is real and what is you. How can I trust you when you put me on high alert no matter the trigger? But the truth is, I feel you respond, react, remove, reassemble... I feel sad when I sense you. I see myself in you. My nine-year-old self. A part of me frozen in time, replaying on repeat. Because it wasn't your fault. I'm sorry I'm so critical of you. I know you are just doing your best to protect me. I know you are just doing what you have existed to do for hundreds of thousands of years. You are the deepest time that lives within me. I think I should probably talk to you more often. Then I can tell you what it is I need. What I needed before isn't what I need now. I'm still figuring out what it is I need now, so I will let you know. How should I talk to you?

Donna

Dear body of parts,

Arms, toes and legs, long and sturdy,
pounding the ground as I run. Hit concrete.

Dear head, who rests on a pillow,
who holds my thinking and stores my pain.

Dearest eyes, who stare into souls, searching for safety.

Dear fingernails, you are getting so long and elegant.
I have changed something in my diet, and you seem happy.
I wish I knew what it was.

Dear stomach, soft, belly, I keep you flat.
I want you strong, you shield me.

Dear ears, pointed flaps, listening out for danger.

Dear neck, strained sinew, tensely alerting me to distant panic.

Body. I love you. I love you. I love you. I write this love song
to you; I write a melody onto your skin. I whisper, I coo. I curl
up and caress. I like you. I starved you. I was ashamed of you.
I wrongfully accused you. My love letter is an apology for how
I have treated you. Shunned you. Punched you. Rejected you.
Shamed you.

Dear toes, I dry between you. I dress you in socks. I put you
in shoes. I let your bare feet touch the sand. I trim your nails.
I paint you.

Dear legs, I shave you. I massage you with a rolling pin.
I stretch you.

Dear torso, I touch you. I let you carry weights.
Your strength, I build.

Dear arms, I hold you. I hug you so tight. I let you explore me.

Dear head, I fill you with knowledge and wisdom
and I let you tell me the hurt of my heart.

Dearest body, separated from me. I respect you.
Forgive me for hurting you.

Khale

A LOVE LETTER

To my thighs. I love that you have become so strong. You've carried me around my whole life, and I've always taken my feelings out on you, but for the first time these last few months I feel like I've been treating you well. Running, walking, stretching, doing squats and lunges, building you up, feeling you get firm and strong. I'm so thankful that you carried me around for all those years even when I hated you.

I'm sorry for everything I ever did to you. Every bathroom I sat in, hunched on a toilet, carving pieces out of you with razor blades or pieces of glass or knives. I cried so many tears into your wounds. Thank you for offering your soft flesh up to me time and time again so that I could get it out, feel my pain, feel grounded again, get out of my head and back into reality. Thank you for all the blood you gave me to bring me back down to earth.

I'm sorry for all the bruises — for the times I hit and scratched you, beating you when I really should have been pushing my anger outward.

I'm sorry for all those marks left on you by predators. Angry blue imprints of grabby fingers and powerful hands. I'm sorry for how often you were forced apart. Thank you, thank you, thank you that every time someone hurt you, you still picked me up and carried me home, walking, riding, running, sprinting, panicking, back behind a locked door.

Thank you to my thighs. You hold me upright on days when I want to fall down. Thank you for all the times you drew up to my stomach and held my quivering guts in. Thank you for curling me into a tight little ball until I felt calm again.

Thank you for being so strong, so capable. Thank you for everywhere you've taken me, and everything you've taken me away from.

Thank you for still responding to a gentle touch, even though you've been hurt so many times.

Dove

All the things I hate and love about me...

All I hate is a painful can of worms. What I love is very little.
I feel I have no right to love anything.

My face, I hate my face. Ugly, disgusting face, stupid features,
boofy hair. Ugly features, I see my father in my face, I hate
it. I hate my skin, containing all the ugliness inside, scarred,
damaged, overly sensitive. Touched, used, abused skin holding
together scarred, damaged insides. Without it I would fall apart,
no longer exist.

I hate my hands, ugly, scarred hands forced to do ugly,
disgusting things, always trembling, giving away my anxiety.

My eyes and expressions, I have no poker face, everything I feel
is written on it. I have been told it causes anger and ire in men.
I have long eyelashes though, I like those.

I am tall, I have mixed feelings. I hated it, it makes me stand out,
it is harder to blend in, to hide. Now I like it, it makes it harder
to stand over or dominate me.

My muscles, I like those, they give me the strength I need
to defend myself. Allow me to run, hit, kick, elbow, and knee.
When I am injured, I find it hard to leave the house. I am more
vulnerable which I can't stand.

My genitals, anything that makes me a woman I hate.
They are the reason I was used and abused.

Claire

ALL THE THINGS I LOVE ALL THE THINGS I HATE

I love the idea of writing a love letter but I hate the idea of writing it to a part of my body. I love the winter sun but I hate the cold hand on my lower back. I love irises; I hate the way they die into themselves. I hate the child that was vulnerable and loving and open and was abused. I love the way children play. I hate anything childlike, I won't wear pink or pyjamas. I hate the sound of lawn mowers and vacuum cleaners. I love the chain of hearts plant, I hate that the chain is broken. I love my solitude, I hate loneliness. I hate people being close to me, I love people being close to me. Part of me just wants to be left alone so I can get on with the business of being lonely. I love being loved. I love being loving. I hate the part of me that pops up every time I am happy with its angry scribbled face saying you don't deserve this. I love water features, I hate dripping taps. I love birdsong in lockdown. I love that the birds love the plane free sky. I love the paintings in my house. I hate I cannot keep a car not looking beaten up. I hate that I drop things, can't hold onto them. I hate cold concrete. I hate being tired all the time, like I live at the bottom of a lake. I love the dark green of bulrushes. I love the smell of earth on my hands. I love the winter sun. I love a cup of tea in the sun in the cane chair in the backyard. I love the smell of herbs. I love the bird shadows that flit across this page as I write. I love the view from this window. I love that I can know that it's what happens now that matters. Fuck the past, the memories. I hate when the past threatens to overwhelm the present. I love being a writer. I love doing a PhD. I love reading. I love my books. I love my friends. I love listening and talking and exchanging ideas and being altered by the ideas of others when my own are like weeds. I love weeding and letting delicate plants see the sunlight. I love my first coffee. I hate my fourth coffee. I love the thought of having breakfast with loved ones. I love cake. I love making cakes.

Reclaiming me | Self-esteem

Julie

Reclaiming my wholeness

Now where do I start

First I must

Listen to my heart

It's beating so fast

As anxiety sets in

Will I sing a song

Of peace within

My words are few

But my mind is light

Please help me make it

Through the night

Donna

A farce. An unrealistic dream, you flat footed fool.
You have nothing to reclaim. So low, so worthless.
What will you reclaim? The truth of dirt. The truth of foulness.
The truth of tortuous thrills? Reclaiming is a desire that seems
out of reach, a desire of delusion.

Dove

I don't even know what that means, what that feels like or looks like. I haven't been whole since I was three. It's like a weird foreign concept beyond my grasp and understanding, like wishing to fly or walk on water. A magical idea that is for others but not me.

Lauren

Reclaiming me feels wrong at first. My brain screams and shames me. But I am reminded by those that love me, who are here with me. Reminded that I matter, that I deserve love and especially self-love. My thoughts calm from their reactive spiral. I can see things again. I find that inner voice, the part of me that will never give up.

Khale

I want to reclaim myself, to love myself. But this body is so disgusting, so used, so broken. It has been treated like garbage by others and by me. I don't know that I am worth saving. I wish I knew how it felt to love myself. But I'm all used up, ready to be thrown away, just a waste of space, I'm garbage, I'm disgusting, I'm dirty. I'm not worth reclaiming. It would be better to start over again with someone new.

Nikki

Reclaiming me — I question my rights and the extent
to which I can. Is it empowerment or white privilege —
can I reclaim myself and not hurt others?

Am I *gaslighting* myself?

Am I hurting others?

I'm afraid and tapped in darkness and uncertainty.
Two parts yell they want safety for us and everyone —
but how is a point of difference.

Julie

Self-esteem is something I lack

Where did it start

I start to look back

I hate myself

For all that I fear

What are others thinking

I try to be clear

Is it my voices

That try to break me down

No self esteem

I can't be that clear

You are this

And you are that

Dove

A tricky concept, something I feel I have no right to.
Something that opposes my programming to serve,
please, submit. I don't know how to stand up for myself,
to achieve it. All I know leads to the destruction of it.

Lauren

I get so envious of people who have high self-esteem.
I hate them for their ease of movement through life.
That they can reach for their potential. I feel like I have
to constantly wade through shit to do that, and then locate
myself in it.

Nikki

I have mixed feelings about my meat sack, my vessel.
The rhetoric of love yourself — can't I just feel nothing?

I have things that I feel positively about myself — I use them
to combat my inner critic sometimes. Like, today my hair
is rocking! In response the voice says "but are you worthy
of respect? You imposter."

Khale

How can someone who has been abused ever be expected
to have self-esteem? We have been treated like dirt, like lowly
animals, used and broken and thrown away. People told us that
we are nothing, worthless, no one will believe us, we are liars,
awful bad children. How can we believe anything different
about ourselves? We have been labelled sinners since day one.
Our bodies are evil. We believe it.

Donna

Self esteem

Out of steam

Running

Self esteem

Is mean?

Self esteem

Is thinking nice things

Is wearing dresses

Makeup

Having nice hair

Being told you are pretty

It's having a bath and feeling slinky

Self-esteem is holding your head high

It is walking into a room and feeling like you've got this.
    Not, I wish I was dead

Gabrielle

Positive sexual experiences and feelings of compassion
    are rare and small.

I don't know what's wrong with me.
    I keep rehashing uncertainty.

Always that I look like shit till the point that I feel
    like shit and am shit.

Studying this semester has been a long journey of fear.

Will I fail this subject?

He / She / They / I pushed... | I turned...

Julie

He pushed and pulled

And threw me to the ground

Only darkness lay all around

The ground was rough

And my body was limp

Who the hell is this person I fear

Out of nowhere

A stranger appeared

Pulled me from behind

As I fumbled for my keys

I looked for a face

But nothing was there

I wish I hadn't worn a skirt in this air

I could feel the rocks

Push into my back

I fought so hard but had to pull back

A very strong hand over my face

This person is a fucking disgrace

My skirt pulled up

And there was no way out

I thought he would kill me

So I didn't move

Nobody came

My screams were unheard

He pushed me down

With such intent

His only thought

Was rape that evening

I felt so disgusting

And when it was over

I lay lifeless

With bruising on my shoulders

I found my keys

And jumped in the car

Not knowing where I was going

Everywhere seemed so far

I finally got home

And showered for what felt like hours

I scrubbed so hard my skin was bleeding

This fucking bastard

What was he thinking

So many feelings running through my head

What do I do now

I wished I was dead

I talked to police

But they weren't really hearing

Too hard of a process

Just go like your dreaming

They shoved me in hospital

A bloody psych ward

Donna

I pushed and gave up a long time ago, as a tiny girl. I knew I had lost the battle. I pushed and I fell over. They pushed and landed on top of me, crushing me, stepping on my lungs, no breath, wind cut through me, sliced frozen hour. I pushed and I screamed to get off me, get the fuck off me, but they taped my mouth, so the sounds were in my head. I lived in my head. I never knew it was important to externalize. Let the pain move through me. A teacher said writing about trauma is externalizing it. I did not know this is what I was doing. Inside my head, I internalized the externalized, I built towns and cities and hid treasures. I held parties. I was successful and dangerous. I was an anime character crossing the threshold of good and evil. I held the keys to the city. I controlled who came in, who got out.

What I really want to say is, what I really want to say is, what I really want to say is, what I really want to say is, I am afraid to speak the inner workings of my mind. I write in my head; essays, books, monologues, but when pen comes to paper, there is a great freeze, as though to tell the truth of what happened to my body and my mind and what I saw, would cause house fires and carnage and be clocked by censorship ratings that don't yet exist. Yet there is power in putting it out there. I know that from early recovery. Standing in twelve-step rooms, telling people that I fantasised about a random stranger walking into the room and shooting me in the head, to relieve me, the more I said it, the less power it held. The more I say it, the less power it holds.

I pushed and pushed and pushed and blacked out because they made me. They laughed at me and said you liar, you made it all up, you live in fantasy. And I accepted it, the internal fantasy inside my head.

Khale

She pushed me to the ground in the middle of a crowded street. She had pushed me before, but always behind closed doors. I didn't know that this was something we did in public. She pushed me down and left me in the gutter, storming away. I had to fix this somehow. I had to fix this here, outside the house, or I knew when we were back in the apartment things would be worse. Things would break, doors would slam, I'd be pushed to the floor and face that familiar choice of letting the anger escalate or enticing her to release her feelings on my body until she calmed down.

She pushed me to the ground that day because she was mad that I wasn't OK. I was at breaking point. I was so suicidal that she believed that I'd already taken an overdose and that she would have to deal with the fallout. She badgered me until I assured her that I hadn't taken anything yet, and then she was so mad at my *drama* that she threw me down there in the street and left me.

Sometimes I wonder what would have happened if I hadn't gone after her. What would have happened if I *had* made an attempt that day and made it her problem to deal with. Would she still have been so mad at me? All those times she took a knife and threatened to slit her own wrists just to torture me, and yet my genuine distress was *too much drama*.

I'm sick of being *too much*. Trying to minimise myself so as not to inconvenience anyone. I'm sorry that I'm like this. I know I shouldn't be. But every time you take your anger out on me, you make it worse. You fracture me a little further. You dial up the crazy, making it that much harder for the next person who tries to help me.

She pushed me to my limit. I finally reached a point where I realised that if I stayed with her, killing myself was my only escape. I still can't believe I got out.

Dove

I turn around and there is fire, bars, snarling, gnashing teeth.
There is no escape, I am trapped in this cage.

Still, I turn desperately, the fire burns, I am terrified.
Dogs are snapping. I back away, fire, it is too hot, the bars
are too hot. Sharp pain, my knees buckle, but I keep my feet.
I turn around, one of them has shocked me with a cattle prod,
I turn, move away, jump back from an angry snarling dog.
It is huge and angry.

The smoke makes my eyes burn. I am beyond terrified,
everywhere I turn is danger, I am panicking. I am being
programmed, terror is a favourite and very effective tool.
I collapse, finally it ends, that part of it anyway.

I stumble out, naked, coughing, relieved it is over for now.
My naked body is draped in silk, I am placed on the altar.
It is time to perform. Other girls come, we must have sex
with each other, must put on a show before the men join in.
I turn around, people in robes, watching, anticipating.

I turn further, the cage and smouldering fire a reminder
to behave, I turn back, the other girls are similarly attired.
Satan's prostitutes.

Nikki

I turned and felt my blood run cold. I turned and saw his shape
darken my doorway — afraid, fearful, chills down my spine —
shooting through my body. I freeze — if I hold still maybe he
won't come in, maybe he won't notice — maybe he'd get bored
and leave.

It's strange — that *freeze* can capture both the feeling
and the lack of movement. Verb and adjective. Descriptive
and yet somehow too inadequate to capture the experience.

I blink and am present again — the memory blended with
the present. I'm confused — is something, someone touching
me now? Giant hands-on arms, clamping, restraining. I turn —
there's no one there.

He's behind me again — I turn — empty space overlayed
with an outline — like the after imprint of looking at a light —
it's clearer if you close your eyes. So, I don't — I stay awake
and stare at the darkness so afraid of the monsters behind
my eyes.

I hold myself and turn — he's always right behind, he's a ghost,
a demon, a nightmare made flesh long enough to hurt, to touch
and then gone, just outside the corner of my eye.

I back to the wall and try to look casual — my logical brain
tells me, "if your back is to the wall, there can't be anyone
behind you." It forces the memories to become that again —
just a memory, the past and passed.

Remember — this is real, I whisper to myself — the wall cool
against my back, the cold air in my nose and lungs. My own
hands clasping my arms — nail dug so deep I've made myself
bleed again. All these tiny scars on my body that I put there
in moments where I froze from fear.

I thought I was going to
It's hard to speak out because | What it takes

Lauren

I thought I was going to be one of those thick-skinned, justice-fighting truth tellers. Tough and bold but kind and caring. I had a vision of myself, owning my life, honouring my life, defending my life. Not backing down. Not putting up with shit. Not allowing people's ignorance or insensitivity or other forms of bullshit to get to me. I want to be this person. I could see this person, feel this person. I embodied this person when I had the epiphany that I wanted to report my abuser to the police. That I wasn't going to be silent, that I would grab this moment with all the strength I could muster and come out the other side empowered, healed, victorious. I knew the realities of the broken system, but I still felt so strongly that no matter what happened it would mean something, that it would take me somewhere better and freer and more powerful and honest. But such is the nature of this journey, of confronting a trauma this deep, that I've been held down underwater and forced to watch, pushed to the brink and further then back, only to plunge deeper, darker, taken to places I didn't know existed, with my arms bound and eyes blindfolded. I thought I had so much experience of this already, that I could manage it. I thought I was going to rise above this cruel joke. Then when I didn't, I was given more shame, more self-loathing and disgust, for failing to take my own determined place. I disconnected. My sexuality has been made something I enact with caution and built-in safety barriers. I don't experience the magic of aliveness with any immediacy. There is always a buffer. Am I now worse off? Sometimes I feel I am. But I know this isn't true. To leave it to lie dormant would only stretch this pain out over the long landscape of my life. At least this way I can get to know it and influence the trajectory.

Khale

I thought I was going to kill myself by the time I was 18. That was my plan. But when I discovered I could push those urges away by raining down a shower of tiny cuts, it seemed less urgent.

I thought I was going to kill myself by the time I was 21. That seemed long enough to have been alive. When I worked in the lab, I snuck in early every day to spend time in the fume cupboard, breathing in every carcinogen we had on hand, praying for God to give me cancer. It didn't work out that way.

I thought I was going to be dead by the time I was 25. I had suffered long enough, surely. I didn't need to keep pretending I wanted to be alive. I got good and drunk, threw myself around a bit, then got on my bike and rode out to the highway. I tried so hard to get in the way of something big — a bus, a truck — but everyone was so good at dodging me. Why were they so determined not to hit me? After trying for a while, I just gave up and went home. Can't do anything right. Or maybe it just wasn't my time.

I thought for sure I was going to end it before I was 29. 30 years is far too long for someone as wretched as me to live. God had made a mistake in letting me go on for this long. It was time. I had suffered enough and forced others to suffer me too. But I calculated wrong, didn't take quite enough pills — stupid, stupid, stupid — and woke up the next day with nothing worse than a hangover.

Somehow, I made it through all these milestones, and to my extreme disbelief, I made it to a place where I no longer plan my demise. I don't foresee my end date anymore. For the first time, I am living instead of just surviving. I can entertain the possibility that I might actually get old, or at least that I might die by something other than my own hand.

I never would have believed this was possible for someone like me. That I could be alive, and happy, and happy to be alive. I still look at myself with disbelief sometimes. I don't know this new person, but I am getting familiar with her. I think she's going to be OK. And no matter what happened in her first three decades, from here on out I think things are going to be good.

Nikki

It's hard to speak out because of the fear. The fear that speaking
will hurt, that I'm telling a story, my story inadequately.
The fear that speaking will hurt me or my family, bring
out a shame, me, into the light. The family secret. I worry
my story will damage them, be misinterpreted.

It's hard to speak out when we were conditioned to stay silent.
The secret, someone else's shame shoved down our throats,
then lips sewn shut — the secret lodged in the throat, choking
us, but left so long we forgot what it was to not have it there.
Until it was normalised, the weight bending me forward,
weighted down.

It's been left so long the skin has grown over the stitches —
and speaking takes the strength to rip it apart — sometimes
I think that has to happen.

By speaking out we can dislodge the secret, the shame,
and throw into the light — start a fire and burn the powerful
liars, the abusers.

I think sometimes

What I really want to say...

What I really want to say...

What I really want to say is that speaking out is scary,
and sometimes, most of the time I don't know if I'm doing
it right. I want to protect, to fight, to stand strong — but this
fucking weight makes it real fucking hard.

I think I struggle with the complexity of the world, of shades
of grey. Of knowing who and when to believe, or protect,
or hide, or run. Is it because I'm broken? Broken into parts?
Or does everyone feel this way — like my centre wants to stand
tall and strong, but my limbs didn't get the memo and are flailing
— it's difficult to feel strong when your limbs are waving,
boneless like noodles.

What I really want to say is I'm ashamed and confused
at how I can help — myself and others.

Dove

It's hard to speak out because no-one wants to hear.
They want to stay in their safe bubble, blissfully unaware
that SRA exists and is happening in their community.

It's hard to speak out because people would rather judge
me in ignorance than hear the awful truth. They prefer
to judge me, label me, disregard me. "But she looks fine,"
"she's just lazy," "time you got over it."

It's hard to speak out because I'm worn down, beaten,
exhausted, battered, and bruised. I have nothing left.

It's hard to speak out because my abusers are powerful people
and cover their tracks well. They have influence, reputations
and "surely could never be involved in such things." I'm just
a fucked-up mess, easy to disregard.

It's hard to speak out because my abuse was so horrific, people
can't bare to hear it. They think and want it to be unbelievable,
claim SRA doesn't exist, my experience isn't real.

It's hard to speak out because of the shame,
disgust and self-loathing, the self-hatred.

It's hard to speak out because of the dissociation
and programming. Even when victims remember,
their brain has been hard-wired to never say a word.
It's dangerous to speak out, you can disappear.

Donna

What it takes is action and courage and denial and love and curiosity and desire and disbelief and revenge and answers and talking and drawing and words and language and writing and exercising and sweating and crying and shaking and howling and dissociating and fighting fear and powerlessness and huddling into a ball and teddy bears and ice-cream and reading other people's stories and twelve-step meetings and stable jobs and painted nails and money and nice clothes and confidence and smiling and laughing yoga and praying and losing sleep and defending and attacking and whispering and dreaming and strength and positive podcasts and late night internet searches and other survivors and stories and feeling and sharing and talking to yourself and reading and laughing and sitting still and breathing and dogs and bathing and intimacy and listening and stopping and starting and nightmares and sleeping and fantasizing and staring and wishing and holding and kicking and screaming and hurling and banging and headaches and stomach pains and icky and scary and remembering light not dark and walking and stretching and being still and keeping clean and makeup and coffee and running and boxing and cloud watching and noticing seasons and courage and denial and hypervigilant arousal and heavy eyes and green tea and books and scholarly thinking and big words and reasoning and ideas and possibilities and imagination and building and noticing small moments.

Intimacy | Effects of my abuse
Write a letter to your inner child
What is meaningful?

Khale

Intimacy is something I've fought so hard for over the years. It felt so impossible to be vulnerable for so long, whether it was emotional vulnerability, or something as simple as being naked.

My first girlfriend had to put up with a lot. The first time she tried to put her hand on my hips or thigh, I freaked out and slapped her away. Back then I didn't even know why I was so upset. I didn't even remember anything. I just knew that there were parts of my body that should never be touched, because bad things would happen. It would hurt. I was scared. I don't know.

She was patient for so long, always asking consent, "is it OK if I put my hand here?" It built such trust between us. But eventually I guess she had waited long enough. We were kissing and she tried to put her hand between my legs. I pulled away, told her to stop, but she put her hand over my mouth and pinned me down with her body, which suddenly felt so big even though she was only a teenager. I felt her hand forced into my jeans, but I don't know what happened after that. That was when I learnt that I would just black out if things got bad, like my brain short-circuited and had to power down.

When I woke up, she was sitting on the end of the bed with her head in her hands. I asked her what happened, and she said "Nothing. You blacked out so we stopped." She wouldn't talk to me for the rest of the day though. I felt a pain down there, but I later learnt that any time I blacked out or woke up from anaesthesia, I would hurt between my legs. I never know exactly what my body is remembering when that happens, because my mind has always shut down when things get bad, to keep me safe. I'm glad I can't remember the worst of it because the flashes I have already haunt me. I wish there was a way to get those feelings out of my body for good, but it's like my insides are scarred and even time doesn't heal the wounds.

Lauren

I always felt a pull towards honesty and authenticity in my relationships. If I met someone who I could share freely with, revealing a person who wasn't striving to look or sound or act like a particular identity, I would latch on. Probably too freely, and not always in my best interest. It gets me in trouble when I misjudge it, when I go in too strong, too soon with someone I barely know, desperately hoping they will reciprocate, that they will participate, and in doing so affirm my own experience, help me feel less alone, less of an imposter, that there are other people like me in the world. I've always struggled with niceties and small talk, even though I can be good at it. I feel like I'm participating in a charade. I don't know where this feeling comes from, but it always has a sense of disconnection, like I am detached from my body, like the person I am pretending to be is not real and that everyone else can see it. I feel lost, floating, directionless. I feel dispossessed. People have always struggled with my need for intimacy and radical honesty. I will point out their flaws at the same time as attempting to forensically examine my own. I am searching for a reason, the truth, salvation. There's no point lying to yourself. I want to see clearly and look at what is really there, examine its clinical ugliness and banality. I want to unpack every argument and identify how a trigger led to an emotion and uncover how our childhoods were placing us to react the way we did. I want your healing to be wrapped up in mine. Is there any other way to heal? But at the end of the day, this freaks people out. It's intense. I struggle to be light and easy-going and spontaneous. I think my seriousness around connection and intimacy is rooted in my need for control, to feel in control. Honestly, I wish I could be less serious. My emotions seem wired this way. It's too much for me a lot of the time. But it's also given me the gift of authentic relationships. I just need to remember to cultivate an authentic relationship with myself.

Dove

The effects of my abuse go on and on,
I will never be completely free of them.

My world view is skewed, my fears are too many to count,
my faith in humanity and self-esteem are non-existent.

The emotional scars are deep and painful. Pain so intense
I had to cut to release it, to cope. The psychological damage
so great my brain broke into parts, too many to count.
I black out, my brain short-circuits like an overwhelmed
power board. DID, BPD (borderline personality disorder),
social phobia, anxiety, depression, complex PTSD, all a result
of 20 years of abuse.

I struggle with identity, who am I? I struggle with disgust,
shame, self-loathing, hatred, all the pain and humiliation
I have to keep reliving in order to process it. I long to die,
to be free of my past, it is likely impossible.

The person I would have been is dead and gone, the chatty,
intelligent little girl with her whole life in front of her died
aged three. She died over and over again over the years until
a shell was left. Cutting, eating disorders, high-risk behaviours
and a death-wish replaced career, relationships, becoming
a mother and an ability for joy, love, and trust. I merely existed,
praying they were finally telling the truth when they promised
I would be dead by 30, unable to cope in the world I found
myself stuck in.

Julie

To my dearest child if you could see me now

My head is in turmoil

And my bodies a wreck

I will write to you

But I will take baby steps

I'm sorry for all the pain

You were put under

It was no choice of my own

You made me shiver each time you groaned

Each touch resembled the pain inside

I couldn't even cry

A poor young girl

Who had her whole future

Just taken away

Each and everyday

How could I stop it all

I felt myself drowning

I didn't want you to feel

What was happening back then

We often stood in the corner

And counted till we reached ten

Foreign objects were thrown around

Which one would they choose

I hover in fright

I tell the small girl please don't be scared.

I'll take the full blunt

So you won't be hurt

The blood would flow

And the pain is as relentless

But I saved that little girl

From going through the obvious

If only I had my own children

I would protect them from what the world gave to me

I would hide them from pain, revolution and a world of misery

Claire

Dear children. I know that when you were in the kitchen and your brother was in the roof, an axe fell through the roof. Was it deliberate? He was in the roof, no one else was around. Men on the roof shouting to each other, plaster is falling. The electricity is being affected. The light is flickering. Big bang now I can see the holes. The holes were always there now I can see sky through them. Emotional sobriety. See the holes, see the sky, it rains inside. Dear child, your hands are in prayer-position. You really did believe. A rosary draped over your hands. I hated you for being so vulnerable. I didn't feel present sitting on the couch with him. I said why don't we sit on the floor and run our hands over each other's faces, he agreed. An exercise in intimacy. Then I said something that upset him and he completely closed and I completely opened and flew from sanity slamming the already slammed door. Dear child people say you can hold her. I hate her for letting herself be abused by being so open and loving. I still can be open and loving. Being loved is more challenging, that angry child screws her face up and screams "you do not deserve love, what are you doing." Dear child I know you are angry that is understandable, but you are not driving the bus right now. You do deserve love dear child it's ok you were loving and trusting I can hold you now protect you. You are held, you are loved. Dear child look at that photo of you, you did exist. Someone who lived across the road from me, from the family home sent me a photo on FB (Facebook) of me and him in a school photo, so young so real. I blocked him, why? I had cut off, forgotten he existed, I existed, confronted with that child as if I had made up not just my abuse but my whole childhood like it didn't exist if I didn't look at it. Dear child you do exist I know you are there dear child. In that white communion dress. No wonder you do not wear white. Nothing to do with pasta sauce. Dear child you were hungry that's not ok, dear child I will not starve you now. I know it's hard to eat hard to swallow but I will feed you cook for you. Food to be enjoyed. I know you can't swallow.

Donna

Dear Parts,

What I know now is that I am, we are,
    survivors, resilient and brave.

I know that feelings cannot hurt us,
    although they feel like they can.

I know that drinking and drugging and sex with random people
is an ill formed coping mechanism that leaves us feeling icky
and disconnected and sick and ashamed.

I know that the abusers are evil, and they spout horrible things
    that are more about them than you all.

I know that exercise is empowering, animals are healing,
and writing is a creative way to re-story ourselves.
I know that art is voice and unconscious truth and freeing.
I know that when you have been hurt and connect with it,
you develop empathy and compassion and there are a lot
of people in our world who need empathy and compassion.
I know that it is safe to listen and draw and play even if it
does not feel like it. I know that love is the answer but needs
to be redefined and a new meaning arrived at. I know that
God loves everyone and is inclusive, funny, and warm hearted.
I know that it is okay to stay in bed all day even if we never do.
I know that telling our story helps others and that we can use
what has happened to us to live a new life, it can inform us,
not break us, it can be a weapon to save us, not destroy us.
I know that darkness is real and there are sick people in this
world, and it is better to accept that rather than deny it because
when we deny it, we perpetuate the lies and I know that it is
okay to trust, but not everybody and it is okay to have your
guard up, but at the same time be open to experience. I know
that life is a metaphor and language is layered and your heart
is alive, real, and safe. Not damaged. And I know that it is
better to live and love in full and sound like a poster art cliché,
than to shut off any potential to grow and be free. And I know
that it is okay to be looked after and to heal you must hurt
even though I have not fully let you do this.

Claire

Making meaning. We make meaning. It is not that it is meaningful or not meaningful. It is about making meaning. Making meaning of freedom is making bikinis out of face masks and dancing in the lounge room with my partner. That is making meaning of personal freedom. Making meaning, making story. Making garden, making sense. Everything has meaning or nothing has meaning, a kookaburra means fidelity, a search engine said so. It doesn't matter if that is true or not if I make it have that meaning. I make meaning out of symbols and dreams. I write myself into this story, this room. I have made this story. What is meaningful? Nothing is meaningful till I give it meaning. I don't know what I think and feel till I make it meaningful. The community is meaning other people see me, their seeing me creates me. My no to their seeing I am not a pawn in other people's play. If I say no I make meaning of the line around my body that is skin of containment. What is meaning making, fun masks, meaning of breaking tension. Take something back as mine.

This is the first time in my life it's easy not to break the law. All I have to do is wear a mask not to break the law. What law was I breaking when I walked the streets and the police pulled me up and asked for my name and address? What law was I breaking asleep in my bed? I broke the law of vigilance, I broke the law of not falling asleep. When I filled in forms for social security as a single mum wrong, I didn't mean to break the law. It's against the law to be poor, I learnt, criminalize being poor, I make meaning of wearing a mask. This is the first time in my life it's clear how to not break a law. But fuck it it feels like a hand over my mouth.

Khale

What is meaningful in these writings? Every week I listen to each person read their thoughts aloud and I feel somewhat out of place. Everyone is so creative, writing poetry and metaphors and weaving stories with their words. I am a biographer at best. I do not know how to write creatively. All I can do is recount my stories. This is what happened to me. This is how I felt. And now this is where I am. Is that meaningful? It's not pretty, it's not poetic. So often my words sound so ugly coming out of my mouth. I wish I could create something beautiful, something worthwhile. Something more than just a laundry list of my traumas, counting them off one by one.

I want my writing to be better, to be transformative. That's not why I came here. I didn't come to this group to become a wordsmith. I came here to work on my history — to expose to the light secrets I've seldom ever spoken before. I don't want to hold these things secret anymore. While I feel ashamed of thrusting all these awful stories upon others, I feel so honoured to have a group of people who I know will hold my stories safe for me. I don't have to carry everything on my own anymore.

I feel lighter now than I did a few months ago. I feel like some of those rocks I always carried around in my stomach have been worn down. They're smaller, smoother, less painful. Still a small, quiet part of me, but not dragging me down so that I know I would drown if I fell in the water.

What I'm really trying to say is, I guess I'm just surprised. I'm surprised that talking about everything that has always made me feel so ashamed can make me feel *less* worthless, *less* disgusting. Like all my words matter, and yet no matter how awful the things I say are, they don't make me a bad person.

Lauren

What is meaningful? Not meandering conversations where no one says what they really mean. Obfuscating dialogue, clashing egos. It is not pretending you know something you don't because you are too arrogant to acknowledge your flaws and human vulnerability. It is not ignoring suffering and paying lip-service, so you look caring. It is not generalising whole communities and generalising pain. It is not being right or revered or honoured, put on a pedestal. It is not taking yourself so seriously that you stop hearing the people around you. What is meaningful is the opposite of laziness, which is not to say it is productivity. Productivity does not create meaning. Purpose matters. My most meaningful moments of revelation and insight have come from moments of complete respite from the wheels of capital, career. What is meaningful is not persona but character. What is meaningful is honest, heartfelt, real. What is meaningful is knowing the reality of our worth and humanity, having a voice and claiming a space. What is meaningful is not stubborn, but a willingness to sit with discomfort and think and learn and grow. I am afraid I will stop doing this. What is meaningful is terrifying, overwhelming, beautiful, if only briefly. Sometimes I don't have a clue what is meaningful. Sometimes the most meaningful act is to admit my own shortcomings, to feel humbled. To claim space is important, but to claim space you have no right to claim is damaging. Knowing the difference is meaningful. What is meaningful is not fixed but exists in a messy landscape of ideas and questions and conversations. What is meaningful is other people, community, and camaraderie.

Trauma

Donna

Blood show shower screen

Woman wake night

Man siren volcano

Hospital surgeon

Scream

Popcorn movies

Police cars

Detective

Taser criminals

Dressing gowns

FANTASY.

Dove

Trauma is all I know, it dominates my miserable existence,
I don't know what life is without it.

I was abused by people whose mission was to inflict as much
trauma and pain as possible on children. They are exceptionally
good at it.

Khale

Trauma seems like such a small insignificant word for something
so big. My trauma is an enormous ball that fills my whole chest.
It comes up my throat when I am just trying to speak.
It is unwelcome, it is always there. People can see it billowing
out of me. I try to contain it so as not to inconvenience anyone.
Not to scare them off.

Lauren

Trauma is a word, a sink, a stink. Too big for one word.
Seems wrong. Makes me laugh. Everyone has it but no one
knows what it is. My trauma. Like it's something I created.

Nikki

Trauma, trauma, where for art thou trauma?

Funny how trauma can be so multifaceted — you don't just
experience it in your mind, but in your body, your limbs,
your stomach, and soul. It's pervasive and ingrained —
layers of sediment turned into stone.

Silence

Julie

It blows quietly through my lips

I can hear in the distance

The echo of a voice

Not realising it is getting closer

I don't want silence

I can hear them approach

What have I got to loose

Just tighten the rope

Hang me from the tree

And there.... once again

We have silence all around

Silence has begun again

Claire

Silence is the inside of rose sleep the red raw of raw
and childlike silence is a blanket of stars silence is cold
is broken silence is fingers around a throat silence is breaking
silence is breaking on rocks is water full breaking ice falling rice.
Silence is in the hand. Silence is contained in an egg in the palm
of a hand silence is soldiered and sorried.

Donna

Silence is stifled breath under water, trapped.

Silence is the way you held me down and zipped my mouth shut, my eyes wide open, covered me in your grime.

Silence is violence, so dangerous the time bomb ticks.

Silence is suffocating and uneasy, it is conversation stilted. It is knowing the truth and feeling as though you cannot do anything about it. Silence is my household.

Dove

Silence is peace. It's freedom from the screams in my head, the screams in my memories, the cruel, biting, soul destroying words, the programming. It's freedom from the insults, taunts, and jeering.

Nikki

Silence is simultaneously comforting and terrifying — it's a state to seek and reject. I need the stillness, the calm, the silence to become calm. But it also terrifies me because of the places my mind may go.

The silence is the antidote to the endless rush of fear and external pressures.

It gives me the space to look within and say, "hello you — I can see you now."

Khale

Silence is evil. You are not supposed to say anything
because people will be upset. Silence is oppressive.
Do you really want to stir up trouble? People will just
say it is your fault anyway. Silence is fucked. Why should
we be silent? Surely, we, more than anyone, are justified
in screaming? I want to shout in their faces. No no no.
It is not my fault. You should have done something. NO.
It is not my fault. Do not tell me to be silent.

Lauren

Silence is stifling, disempowering, consequential.
Silence serves the people with power and silences their
victims. Silence is shame and isolation and victim-blaming.
Silence is never quiet, but controls us all with its towering
shadow, like a monster on the wall of a childhood bedroom.

Writing + Boxing =

Claire

Writing plus boxing equals body memories writing is wading through water going deeper and deeper immersion in mud. Breathing through a straw underwater. Boxing is in the body this body boxing out of body overextending sinking sorry.

Lauren

Writing + boxing = a whole body mind experience.
A recalibration and reminder of my ability to heal and grow. It is the radical expression of my truth, a confrontation of my deepest fears. It does not feel comfortable.

Donna

Writing + Boxing = smash words on pillow paper

Beat down selves

Unconscious connection

Deep seated feelings

Erupted onto paper

Turn into sweat

Drip down body till exhaustion sinks in

Pain on paper

Pain, left, write, hook.

Khale

Writing + boxing = a combination that I never knew could be so healthy. I get stuck right inside my head, but then I get out, out, away, punching, swearing, yelling! My body is my own, my body is strong, my body can fight and protect me. I am not inside my trauma anymore. I am in my body, and it is the body of a fighter.

Nikki

Writing + Boxing = Confidence. Strength. Release. Crescendo.

Writing + Boxing = Exposure. Moving forward, holding space. Hyperventilating on the floor. Crying. Screaming.

Completeness and cycle; connection and finally calm.

Gabrielle

My father took my brothers to boxing early in the morning.

I was never taught to box.

To write your vulnerability then to box to hit to smash your anger to be physical and active where in the past you were victimized.

ROUND THREE

About Round Three

Donna

Round Two explored boxing as a form of recovery-oriented practice. In Round Three, I became interested in the idea of developing and maintaining the physical and mental practice of writing and boxing as a commitment to self. Healing and recovery are not one-off events, they take time, and they are individual processes. Whether writing and boxing becomes the outlet for the survivor is unimportant. Each survivor must find what works for them and allow each practice or modality to develop and mature.

Prior to this workshop round, I undertook a level one intensive in Narrative Therapy. I learnt about the concept of externalising problems (shifting deeply held beliefs from inside self to outside self to encourage a different viewpoint). I began to question how I was tricked into believing lies about myself. I used questions common to narrative therapy practice as prompts from which to write. I became drawn to the concept of (re)storying constructions of our selves through the creative and physical practice of writing and boxing. Although in many ways, this is what I may have been doing from the start, the process evolved as I continued to mature this thinking and formulate my own artistic and professional practice throughout the workshops.

The reader may note that at the beginning of each round, I top and tail the workshops with similar prompts. In each workshop round, I prompt participants to consider why they are here, why they have returned and what it means to come back. I close the workshops, asking the participant to think about what the last eight weeks has meant for them. Sometimes there are great shifts, other times not so. The process is less about transformation. Rather, it is about finding meaning and creativity through (re)claiming narratives and recognising personal inner worth.

Round Three Writing Prompts

I return | This time
I feel | Developing a practice

My commitment to self is
Trusting myself | Trusting others

I was told | Ways I was trained to be powerless
Ways I have reclaimed myself | Feeling powerful

Things I've felt responsible for
My reality | The way I see things

I see you | When you see me
I hear you

Rage | I am angry

Being there for others | In its place | On the way

I pretend | I was tricked
Don't disturb

Preferred ways of being | Prescribed ways of being

The Unknown | The Atmosphere

I say goodbye to | The last eight weeks

Choose one prompt at a time from each grouping above.
Turn your timer on for 10 minutes and write non-stop using
the prompt as your starter line.

I return | This time | I feel
Developing a practice

Khale

I return because I am not *there* yet. I have not arrived. I like to imagine a time and place when I will be free from haunting memories, free from symptoms — no more flashbacks, no more nightmares, no more hating myself for things that weren't ever my fault. Yesterday I watched a video of my old choir singing "I can't keep quiet," the song that became the rallying cry of the #metoo movement, and I broke down in tears. Then last night my wife had to wake me up from a nightmare — I dreamt I was being sexually assaulted by Tony Abbott (former Australian Politician and 28th Australian Prime Minister), which is a kind of fucked up I can't even begin to address.

So, I have not arrived yet, and that is why I am back. This is hard, but it is helping. This is exhausting, but it is helping. This is dragging every sad, shameful, broken feeling out of my body one by one, holding it up to the light, accepting it, and setting it free. It is helping.

I come back each week a little afraid of what I will unearth, how I will feel in the week afterwards, but I know it is progress. It hurts, but it helps. It wears me out, but it helps. Each week I feel like I am one tiny child step closer to feeling peace — peace with all that happened, peace with myself. Maybe peace is the wrong word. I'm allowed to still be angry. But accepting what happened doesn't have to ruin me. That I can still be a worthwhile person, even after everything. That I'm not forever tainted, irreparably broken, not worth saving.

I have value. I have worth. I am creeping closer, week by week, to accepting myself and being gentle with the person I am. She did her best. She is not all bad. She is a person. She has worth. She can still mean something to the world, even this late in life. She is loved. She is needed. She is wanted in deep and intimate spaces. She has something that the world needs.

It is OK that she is still here, still alive. She is supposed to be. It is not a mistake that she has survived this long. It turns out that she belonged in the world after all, that nothing she did or experienced was ever meant to doom her to destruction.

Julie

I return because I have some unfinished business

I return because my story needs to be told

I'll watch my emotions

And I'll try to uphold

I'll walk the path

Where life may lead me

And follow my heart

From here to eternity

I return because I want to learn

Learn the techniques

Of writing, boxing and more

In every direction

I come out wanting more

I know I am anxious

And my heart beats so fast

I'll try my best

And hope this time

I will last

I commit my whole self

To whatever comes up

And follow the direction

Only my heart will know

Tears, anger, frustration and more

I'll buckle down

Till my body can take no more

I feel fitter inside

But I know it takes time

Time to catch up

Especially with boxing

I need to be gruff

Don't feel self-conscious

I tell myself now

But the fear inside

Hopefully will show me how

How to be stronger

And let my defences down

Don't be ashamed

There are people all around

I'll make a connection

With my body and soul

Wanting desperately

To one day just be whole

I return because I love it so much

Even though I am quiet

I am starting to trust

Not just myself

But others all around

Hopefully one day

There will be no shaky ground

Donna

This time I embrace the unknown, I say I am going to listen
to myself and I've never done that before. I've never been able
to listen to myself because I usually hear little voices that tell
me I am scared, that I am covered in blood, they're hurting me.
I'm dying.

This time, I have been soothing them, saying "there, there,
you're safe now, it's okay now." This time I am stronger,
but I am weaker because I accept my weakness.

A ball of hay, buried in it.

This time I am considered, yet beat myself up for being
inconsiderate, as though forgetting is a sign of my damage.

This time, it is hot. This time, the apartment is messy.
This time I am nervous and still ashamed. This time,
I am quietly more confident, but quietly afraid that
I am cocky and crazy.

This time I am focusing on breathing.

This time it's about my body.

I remember my third fight. I was so disconnected from
my body. I just had to remember the punch combination,
that's all I had to do, I said. Next time, I'll work on connecting
with my body, on thinking about my body, as though I had
accepted that my mind and body were two separate phenomena.
I never considered I was already in a body.

So used to standing outside of myself. So used to escaping.

To be in a body meant I was going to feel the pain.

This time I say *go gently*. I hear other survivors say
these things. I steal their words. They resonate.
What does it mean to *go gently*? To be kind to me?

This time, the program kicked into action. I was running,
two weeks back and I could feel the dissociation. I thought
of *Left/Write//Hook*. I began to soothe myself, think about
what I was going to do that was self-care, nice to me,
I stopped running and walked. I felt more connected.

Khale

This time I will be in my body, but conscious of my body.
This time I won't just go as hard and fast as I can, so I don't
have to feel anything. This time I will try to be present.
This time I will listen to my body. This time I will be better.
This time I will be thankful to my body. This time I will be
gentle. This time I will listen. This time I will be a whole person,
not just a ball of fury.

Julie

This time I will allow myself to fall

This time I will always feel my heart

I will rise and fall

In which order I recall

It doesn't matter

The obstacles that may stop me

I will always be

Honest and uphold me

This time I will give it my all

Gabrielle

I feel my dreams. I had a nightmare about my brother.
In the nightmare he said I didn't know how to love.

When I woke it was early in the morning.

For some strange reason I rang the police and told them
what happened with my brother.

The police wanted to know what the call was about.

I replied that I felt embarrassed,
that it was about childhood sexual abuse.

I was put onto a female sergeant; her last name was like a wine.

She said I had to contact the police station
where the abuse took place.

She said she would get back to me but never did.

So I rang the sexual offence unit where the abuse took place.
I mentioned the female sergeant and said that no one got
back to me.

I had to describe my abuse to a male senior constable.
He asked me if I wanted to make a statement.

I said I did.

The constable rang back once and said he would again.

The police officer who took the statement about what happened
with my brother was compassionate and understanding
about the abuse.

I feel estranged from my family,
unsure if I should even communicate with them.

Lauren

Developing a practice means we are setting up an alternative
scene. A site of resistance and survival against the systems
that don't serve us. A place where we together are reminded
of who we really are; our intrinsic worth. Our power and resolve.
It is radical. It makes me feel free. It does not come easily.
But my awareness of its importance makes me keep going.

My commitment to self is
Trusting myself | Trusting others

Nikki

My commitment to self is a slow journey and growing relationship. It's steps forward and back, making mistakes, taking a break, but always returning and trying again.

My commitment to self is setting boundaries with loved ones and keeping them. Sometimes they might look like a ribbon — that eases and tenses with need. But others are a stone wall, high and long as the great wall of China — immovable and a strong wonder of the world.

It's building communication with the parts of myself — being curious and learning about each of them. Not all of my parts are always easy to love or understand — but the commitment I make is to trying. It's also about respecting their boundaries and knowing that sometimes they might lock me out — for my protection or theirs.

My commitment to self is unlearning and re-teaching — replacing old patterns with new habits. It's woven of compassion, resolve and solace. It might fray or come apart, but as long as the elements remain, I can begin again.

My commitment to self is defining where I end, and the world begins. It's about knowing myself better and committing to my own rehabilitation. A reminder that even burned woodlands recover — green sprouts out of the charred earth and trunk. It may be different, but it endures.

My commitment to self is knowing my weaknesses and deficiencies and loving myself anyway. It's about being kind.

What I really want to say is…

What I really want to say is that

What I really want to say is that I feel that I need to define boundaries or limits to myself — a golden outline that surrounds me — radiating its own light. I feel when I have that, then I can ride these seas of change — of other's emotions. Rise and fall without it drowning me.

Donna

To show up

To listen

To breathe

To punch away negativity

To ground

To cry

To laugh

To practice

To accept mistakes

To breathe through chaos

To breathe

To breathe

To feel the ground

To feel moving

To move

To practice moving

To feel the hurt

To acknowledge the pain

To tolerate the discomfort

To talk about the discomfort

To remember many other women have gone before me

To remember I am not alone.

Lauren

Trusting myself feels so new. There is probably no more reliable feeling in my life than my distrust of myself. But more than that, a deeply held fear that everyone else knows something I don't. I think I trusted the world around me a bit too much because of this. What I'm really trying to say is I was sceptical of anything self-generated. I looked to others for cues of how to be and how to act. I sought approval from everyone and everything. If I held a belief and there was a dissenting belief, expressed with conviction, by anyone, anywhere, I felt lost, like there was nothing solid that I could hold onto, that I could lean on. That I was too stupid to understand why I was wrong. That's at the heart of it really. An underlying feeling of wrongness that followed me everywhere, reminding me that my opinions were ill-informed, or my clothes were embarrassing or that my body was gross. It's a powerful force for action. It's what drove me to lose so much weight that I lost my periods. I've realised that this is shame. And through realising this I am beginning to understand that shame is a motivating factor behind many of the things I have done to construct a life. My high standards at work, and my willingness to work myself to the bone to succeed, essentially is a process of identifying and eliminating anything that would open me up to criticism or reveal that I'm an incompetent failure. My perfectionism, obsession with detail, order, cleanliness, control. All these things have been positively reinforced by the world around me because they look good on paper: good grades, a functioning life, impressive professional outcomes. But to me, my experience of achieving these things was/is existential. Not achieving them is not an option. It's not something I can consider without being overcome by a deep feeling of self-loathing and failure, of having my wrongness proven to me. People see me from the outside and wonder where I find my drive, my intrinsic motivation. But what they don't know is I feel like I'm being held on the edge of a cliff the whole time, desperately working against the urge to throw myself off. It's weird looking back at everything I've managed to achieve and see that it was under duress.

Gabrielle

I cannot trust others. Most of my *friends* are toxic. My *friends* say I am mad, weird, eccentric, sexually unattractive, asexual. They tell me to *fuck off* sometimes as a joke sometimes seriously. Like in pop culture I guess I am the uncool girl that cool girls tell to *fuck off*. They treat me like this, and I send them my books of poetry for free. I cannot rely on anybody. Hell is not other people, it is panhandling in Carlton. When the female comedian gets on the stage, she ridicules my sexuality and the cool guy laughs. When I read a poem about how I was raped the cool guy laughs. When I read a poem about how I was abused in the street for being overweight a woman laughs. FUCK YOU ALL.

Claire

Trusting others, trusting myself, what is that? What is trust, that people, things can be relied on where would that come from? I trust myself that I will have the best intentions not to be reactive no matter what the provocation but I know that everyone including me has their limits. The sun shines, flowers come out, I am lied to, I feel bad. What is the world with no trust there is no trust, what is trust what does it even mean? Is it hope that things I don't want to happen won't happen? What is trust, a handrail, a safety net, what is trust, integrity certainty, love, and commitment, what is trust? Have I ever felt it, have I ever held it, I trust the glass will hold water, glass by its nature breaks, glass breaks, but for a moment it holds water while I bring it to my mouth and miss my mouth or drop it, it slips from my hands. But I trust that the intent of the maker of the glass is that it will hold water until it breaks. What is trust, stability, security? What is trust? Family and institutions that were set up to be a base were not. I was taught to trust untrustworthy people. What is trust? I trust myself but only when I am by myself, only by myself do I feel trust. Is trust safety? I don't know what trust is, is it red, is it a closed window, is it an open field, is it standing under a roof sheltering from the rain, the roof keeps the rain off, is that trust? Trust that I won't betray myself, I don't have that around other people. I have it by myself. Trust others won't betray me, I've never had that, is it self-perpetuating. Trust that this is real, I don't have that. How can I learn something from no basis? What is trust, an abstract concept? A thing not attached to anything, a state of being with no evidence or facts. Just trust regardless. Like sunshine, it's not there all the time but it is still a thing, what are its components, where does it come from. Sunlight comes from the sun, where does trust come from, is it divine, this thing in the face of impermanence and ever changing ground. Everything comes into being and then dissolves, all things come into being exist then don't exist anymore, or has everything that existed still existing, just changed forms. The fact that things finish does not prove that they don't exist. Trust being broken does not mean it is not a thing.

I was told | Ways I was trained to be powerless
Ways I have reclaimed myself
Feeling powerful

Dove

I was told not to tell, or my mum would leave us, my brothers would be hurt, that I was bad, dirty, sinful, I needed to be punished. I was told I am disgusting, that God is angry with me, that I am only good for one thing.

I was told God wanted me to please men, it was my calling and job, that He was disappointed in me because I didn't want to. That I had to make men make the mess or I hadn't pleased them, and God would be angry.

I was told I was a dirty little slut as my face was pushed into the mattress and I couldn't breathe, unbearable weight on my back, crying and screaming muffled because this client hadn't paid for anal or to be so rough. There were other girls who men could pay to mess up. But he wanted me. I was told I was dirty and that I better get used to it because it's my job now and I'm a good little earner. He said he may as well have a go while he waited for me to stop bleeding so I could go back to work.

He told me I had to behave myself as he lay on my face and I choked on his penis. He laughed as my head slammed into the wall as he raped me. Get used to it. I was nine.

They said I wasn't allowed to show pain or scream. I had to pretend to like it, or they'd hurt me worse. They said this video will bring in the big bucks. They said it was a little slut video. I had to pose and smile or else they'd turn really nasty. Then they put the cloth over my face and poured water over it, so I felt like I was drowning while they raped me. I was tied up and sodomised. I realised the building was empty, it didn't matter if I cried or screamed, it was now a rape video. Dad told me to shut up and stop snivelling as I continued to cough up water as he led me out of the building. I was 14.

Julie

I was told you'll never achieve

I was told you'll never be believed

I thought back to those days

When I was living in a haze

A haze that was filled with shame and uncertainty

What was going to become of me

I would shiver and shake

Only to be told you'll never elate

I was down on my knees

Begging please

Please make it stop

Never call the cops

I wanted to run

And escape these demons

I wanted to fly

And soar to the sky

I wanted to be locked up

When I thought I would never be safe

Never understanding what jail really meant

I wanted to be free

And hide the real me

Those bastards they took so much

And to this day

It haunts me so much

They are in my dreams

And it all seems so real

I remember each place

And the secrets that were kept

Kept with me for so long

It's only now I feel strong

Strong is a word

That fills me with so much anxiety

I was tortured so much

It will never escape me

I want the world to know

I'm not that little girl any more

But my body still feels

And it was so sore

They made me do things

I couldn't comprehend

It's only now I finally see an end

In so many places

They took so much

How did nobody notice

When they were all around

I ask myself to this very day

How my life would be

If they didn't abuse me that way

I am still scared

Of so many things

Even the dark

I can never be alone

Not feeling safe

Even in my own home

I walk down the streets

Always looking back

Am I being followed

Down this lonely track

The nightmares come and go

But I'll never escape

My memories from so long ago

Hopefully now the time will come

And maybe soon

They'll rot in that jail

That I once dreamed of

So long ago

It won't be me in there

It will be them

It's not a safe place

Especially for these kind of men

Claire

I was told I was born bad. I was told people are basically evil. I was told people can't control their urges. I was told if a man is alone with a woman and doesn't feel sexually then he must be a cabbage. My father who had five daughters told me that. I was told if you can't say anything nice then don't say anything at all. My mother told me that. I was told I would end up in the gutter. My father told me I was his responsibility till I became the responsibility of my husband. I told him well I'll never marry. I told myself I'll always be alone. The only way to be safe is to be alone. I was told I would go to hell. I was told the only purpose in life is getting to heaven. I was told people are basically bad. I was told not to provoke my brother. Everyone was told not to provoke my brother. I was told he is a softie really. I was told "gee that girl is big boned." I was told to keep my legs together while sitting. I was told I'd end up in the gutter. I was told everyone has their cross to bear. I was told to stay still while I stood on the table in taffeta while my mother pinned the seams. Stuck pins into me. I was told to keep the peace. I was told I had a complex. I was told I wasn't hungry and I had had plenty to eat. I was told

Khale

I was told that she was asking for it. Didn't she know that good girls don't go out with boys without a chaperone? I was told that these things don't happen to good Christian girls. They happen to sluts, to sinners, to girls who knowingly put themselves in harm's way.

Then I was told, no, it's your body that's the problem. Yes, you are good Christian women, but your bodies, you see, your bodies are a walking, breathing temptation. Men, good Christian men, if they see too much of your bodies, they will fall into sin. We mustn't lead men into sin with our bodies. We mustn't be temptresses, Jezebels.

I covered up, always. I was a good Christian girl. I never showed my shoulders, my legs, my chest. I did not want to lead men into sin. But more so, I did not want to invite men into my body. My body. No one ever talked about our bodies being our own. They were these detached, sinful things we just steered around, trying to prevent them from breeding evil.

I never showed my skin, but somehow, men still saw me. It was like they could see through my clothes. They knew I was hiding giant breasts under there. I was so ashamed. I never asked for this body. So, I starved it. I ate nothing for years until there were no breasts left to speak of. But somehow my new, tiny body still triggered something in men. Here is someone so small, so powerless, I could do anything to her. This tiny, weak girl. It is just so easy.

They told me I should have said something. "Why didn't you go to the police?" They also said "This is only going to reflect badly on you. It's your word against his. Do you really want all that attention?"

I was a good Christian girl. I politely declined. I never screamed, I never hit, I never tried to embarrass them. I thought maybe I could just quietly escape using only manners. I never made a fuss. I was demure; I was good.

I was told that these things don't happen to good Christian girls who dress modestly and stay away from dark alleyways. So where did I go so wrong? What horrible deeds did I commit in a past life that landed me with this sinful body that was a walking target?

Donna

I remember terror and fear. Walking on eggshells.

My father was domineering.

We were so scared of him.

I used my charm to soften him, I wanted him to be nice,
I knew he could be nice, I worked so hard to make him nice.

I was trained to be powerless by feeling I could not talk back;
I could not express an opinion or alternative view without it
being shut down.

Told I was ugly, stupid, worthless, disgusting, it was all my fault,
I was a filthy, dirty slut.

I was trained to be powerless.

To believe it was my fault, I had no self-worth. I made it happen.
They gave me the power, yet I was a child, I had no power,
I was powerless, and they reinforced that having any agency,
any power was a bad thing, because look what happened
when I had it! Look what happened when I exercised my power
— it was for evil! All lies. I was trained to be powerless, to accept
lies and not challenge dominant paradigms, to accept what was
happening.

I was trained to be powerless by death threats and silencing
and forgetting.

So later, I led a life of secrets, a double, triple life, everything
segmented, compartmentalized, acting out shame, accepted
by some, consensual with some, no-one ever had a full picture
of me. I split too many times for a full picture.

I was trained to be powerless by being forced and tortured
to totally believe the messages that I was bad, evil and no good.

I was trained to be powerless by watching my sister get beaten,
my mother a slave in the kitchen, by being made to feel like
a burden; guilty.

The ways I was trained to be powerless was to forcibly accept disconnecting from my body, so that feeling anything was a negative. To come into my body was the most disgusting, vile experience I could face. They did that to me.

I was trained to be powerless by not being able to think for myself, by drinking and drugging and believing I should be a prostitute or sex slave or beaten or humiliated. I was trained to be powerless, so I would never speak out, lash out, breathe properly, tell the story, reclaim the darkness. I was trained to be powerless through electrocution and drugging.

Khale

My mum was a good Christian woman. All she ever wanted was to raise good, God-fearing daughters who would grow up going to church, meet and marry a nice Christian man and live less than five minutes away with grandkids.

She trained me to be the kind of girl that could fit that mould. Be polite. Be demure. Don't make a fuss. When my older brothers would wrestle me, she taught me *explicitly* not to fight back. Girls aren't allowed to punch or kick boys because if you accidentally hurt them between the legs, their lives will be over. Don't fight back.

My mum sent me on a date when I was 14. I didn't know it was a date until I was sitting in the McDonald's carpark and she was forcing lipstick on me. Why? Why was it so wrong that I didn't want boys to touch me?

When I was 15, I told mum about what was happening at work. The teenage boys, they make jokes about us, they come onto us, they try to touch us. Mum said "You're being too sensitive. Boys will be boys." I learned that mum would never believe me when it came to boys.

When I was just a kid — six, seven, eight, nine — there was a man at church that none of us liked. He always wanted to hug us. He held on for too long. All the mums told us every week to let him hold us — he was a good Christian man who just wished he had children of his own. When I told mum that he hugged me under my clothes, she didn't believe me. Then when he was convicted, all the mums spoke condemningly as though they had known it all along.

When I was 13 my mum said I had to share a bed with my 14-year-old cousin because we couldn't all fit. I told her I didn't want to because he was a boy and it felt wrong. She actually smacked me on my behind and told me to stop being bratty. I thought I was too old to be smacked.

Every time I raised my voice, tried to stand up for myself, for my body, for my boundaries, I was told *no, no, no*. Be quiet.

Be polite. Don't be too sensitive. Do as you're told. Hug him. Sleep there. Go with him. Let him hold your hand. Appreciate the attention. Flirt back. Men are a prize, and you must always be trying to win them. The goal is to belong to a good Christian man who will take care of you. But all I ever wanted was to take care of myself.

Julie

There are very few times

I have reclaimed myself

Always being what society said was right or wrong

I always felt so very wrong

Not in my body

But what others said was not ok

My sexuality was always frowned upon

But I know in my heart

It was so very right

I always presumed

I had to do the right thing

In other people's eyes

Sacrificing me as a whole being

I feel like I have only reclaimed myself once

Lauren

Times I have reclaimed myself

When I chose to go to art school. When I chose to seek help.
When I faced up to the memory. When I made the complaint.
When I remembered I can choose. When I decided to live
according to my values and stop trying to fit some other mould.
When I wrote about my cancer. When I decided to try boxing.
When I quit my job. When I spontaneously travelled to
Mallacoota with a beautiful new friend I barely knew.
When I decided I deserved to be in a good relationship.

Khale

Ways I have reclaimed myself

I don't know if I have ever reclaimed myself. I guess in
all these years of eating disorder recovery. But I was never
in control then. I was a shitshow. Maybe the times I ran.
Made my body my own. But it still doesn't really feel like
my body. It's just a thing. A thing I hate and fight against.
I wish I didn't have to have a body. At least not a woman's body.
Why can't I just exist as a person without a gendered shape?
Why do people have to see me as a woman first?

Donna

I read last night therapy is a political act

Going to therapy

Drama classes

Performance studies

Finishing a book

Sunbaking without fear

Sex

Laughing yoga

Recovery

12 steps

Leaving 12 steps

Experiencing love

Education

Completing tasks

Running a half marathon

Amateur boxing fights

Setting goals and achieving them

Getting promoted

Sobriety

Having fun

Left/Write//Hook

Saying I am a survivor

Saying it is not my fault and believing it.

Julie

Feeling powerful is unnerving

Feeling powerful is not how I'm feeling

I know deep inside

There's something in me

But it seems hard to see

I do the work

Then come crashing down

Is it worth it

I ask to the clouds

I have always felt

Powerless and weak

Everyone always takes something from me

Why do I let this happen

I don't feel so strong

And have I really been fearless for so long

I decided to take the next step

And suck up the courage

To regain power again

I questioned my thoughts

And my actions too

I won't let any of my hard work

Come crashing down on you

I feel scared inside

But on the outside, I seem strong

What they did was so totally wrong

I took all my tools

And headed down the track

Knowing so many people

Had my back

I held my head high

And walked into the station

I sat in a huge chair

And looked around with trepidation

He was so very kind

And my words just flowed

Everything came flooding back

My voices were loud

And so very confronting

But I soldiered on

Just pushing through my life

I made my statement

It took so long

But everything made sense

I feel so strong

Feeling powerful

Has finally come

I tell myself it's halfway done

The next step is the hardest

To face them alone

To stand in the dock

I need a backbone

So many thoughts

Go running through my head

Different scenarios

Thank god I'm not dead

I play it all out

But who really knows

What will happen

Tomorrow only knows
Will the judge be fair
And hear the real truth
These fucking bastards
Their time will come
I see some light
At the end of the drum

Things I've felt responsible for
My reality | The way I see things

Claire

I felt responsible for the broken bird in my hands. I felt responsible for the broken bird of my sister in my hands, carried up a mountain of crumbling rock. I felt responsible for the broken bird of self in my hands, was it me, was it other. I felt responsible for the closed door and the sounds behind it. I felt responsible for the *it* of my life. I felt responsible for the weather and the pandemic. I felt responsible for the empty car park. I felt responsible for the lift well, losing my car, not knowing which door, getting lost in a shopping centre, not being able to find the exit, not seeing in the dark, not breathing in the dark, I felt responsible for the silence. I felt responsible for the cloud of fog, I felt responsible for not hearing for not seeing for blocking my ears, for not hearing, I felt responsible for chanting so I could not hear the thoughts the words, I felt responsible for what happened, I felt responsible for what happens, I felt responsible, it was me, not them, I felt responsible for the bird call, for the slammed door, for the denial, for not remembering, for forgetting, for everything and everyone, I felt responsible for the crack running along the wall, the marks on the ceiling, I felt responsible for my father, for my mother, for every angry man in every angry situation, the screaming the looks the backward glances the time moving on and around I felt responsible just me if it's just me, feeling safe is not safe, I felt responsible, But if it's just me, just me, pull the cloak around me, just me, the aloneness is safe, close down, shut down, then safe, then sorry, you will be sorry they said, if you don't learn this time you will do it again they said, I felt responsible, stay out of their way, yes that's a good girl, do as they say, appease their anger, you are not like the others you can make it better, you are the only one, you are the only one, that is what made me feel responsible, you are the only one, but if you turn on me I will punish you for all the other ones they said, I will not be able to help it if you can't fix me they said, you are responsible for my violence they said. Fuck them. I am responsible for myself, I am responsible for myself, I am self-responsible, I am self-supportive when you do not support me, I support myself, I am responsible for myself, I am responsible for myself, not then, I could not be, but now, I am responsible for myself, I ask help from those that can and will give it willingly, I am responsible for being kind to myself, to looking after myself before looking after others. I am responsible for rest and recreation for myself, I am responsible for looking up at the sky seeing its blue today, enjoying the garden the birds the things I have grown.

Julie

My reality is a reality

I feel so hopeless

And my life can be a mess

My head starts spinning

And I try to find the beginning

When did it all start

Will I find it in my heart

It started back when

When I was a child about ten

The games they played

And manipulation was laid

I made some friends

Who wanted nothing

But a friendship

And innocent love

As time passed me by

I never really understood why

Why were they so interested

In the way that I looked

I never went out of my way

To look a certain way

I wanted to lay cobbles

And climb all the trees

But their brothers always made me

Made me go down on my knees

I made up stories

Why I was always late

As I was always running, to get through the gate

I tried in my head

To believe it wasn't happening

But everyday was the same

And I couldn't escape

Reality hit when they said I was pregnant

How could this happen

I hadn't even reached puberty yet

I banged on my stomach

So, it didn't feel real

How do I explain

Everything seemed so surreal

Eventually the time came

Finally, I would escape

The cruelty everyday

I made some new friends

And I trusted them wholly

They led me down the track

To a pristine beach

Only to be jumped on

By men out of my reach

They pushed me down

And I stopped counting at ten

Where were my friends

I could hear them laughing out loud

The initiation began

To be part of their group

How low do people really stoop

I lay lifeless on the sand

How could this happen again

Fuck, is there something wrong with me

What's with all these men

This time was different

I decided to tell

As I walked back up the path

I was late

So, I rang the doorbell

My dad answered and let me in

I wanted to say something

But then the beating began

Just because I was late

Sometimes I hated this man

Dove

My reality is ugly, full of darkness and pain. My reality is that I never stop hurting, the pain never ends, the damage is too great. Mind, body, and soul have been completely destroyed, there is no way to fix me, only patch me up so I look and act normal on the outside, fit into other people's reality which is so different from my own.

My reality is monsters, evil and darkness. I know monsters are real, they don't hide under the bed, they get in it. You see them, feel them, fear them, and eventually submit to them. They walk among others like regular people, hiding in plain sight, two alternate realities colliding with regular people none the wiser. My reality is best kept hidden, it has no place in polite society.

My reality is I will never be well, or whole or normal. No-one is supposed to experience what I have and survive. I am dead in so many ways. I don't know joy, happiness, hope or love. Hate, pain, terror and fear are my loyal and constant companions, the devil I know. My reality is I hate them, they run around carefree, pillars of society, committing acts so evil and vile people can't stand to consider the possibility they are real. It's easier to dismiss the fucked-up mess, go back to your corner, sell your body, die, continue to be a toy, just do it quietly. Keep sick fucks happy so we can continue to turn a blind eye to the dark sides' existence.

My reality is hell, I can't stand the sight of myself, my body is damaged and broken, my mind shattered into too many parts to count. I can't function. The normal life that so many take for granted is unattainable. I struggle, fight, fail over and over, the classic example of insanity. I should know better. My reality is that for some reason I am unable to stop fighting no matter how much I want to.

Khale

The way I see things has changed so dramatically. There was some awful news on the Vic Police website for my little community — a man has been frequenting our green space and publicly masturbating. Actually chasing women and girls as he does it. His activity so far has been localised to precisely the stretch of creek that I walk along every day. I know that if I had read this news a few years ago, even six months ago, I would have made an immediate decision — I won't visit the creek anymore. I will just have to give up nature walks.

But not now, not this time. The police report said the man is 165cm tall and slightly built. That's smaller than me. And I am *strong* now, I am fast. I run, I do weights, I do boxing classes. I punch hard and fast.

It was so strange, but as I walked by the creek this week, I found myself thinking *I hope I see him. Let him be here!* I will chase him down and video him with my phone. I will capture his face and then everyone will shame him. If he tries to chase me, I will punch him in the face! I will knee him in the groin! I walked along the creek getting more and more carried away in my head with how much I wished I could confront this sex pest and show him that I wasn't afraid.

This is so different for me. I have always felt afraid. I have always hidden inside when I sensed danger. But I feel so different now — in my mind and my body. I am so physically capable now — I work in the garden with my wife, and I can dig for hours and lift heavy loads and I have so much stamina. I run for miles. I picture people's faces and I punch and punch and imagine breaking bones. And my mind is stronger. I know how much I have survived. I know I am resilient. I have proven time and time again that I can recover from sadness, from hurt, from depression and anxiety and wanting to end it all. I have survived so much, and it has made me strong.

I realised this week when I learnt about our local sex pest that I didn't immediately think of myself as a victim — I thought of myself as strong, as smart, as able to look after myself.

I was determined, not afraid. I was angry, not intimidated. I was ready to fight, not desperate to hide.

This change must have happened gradually over the last six months and I can't believe it. I don't even know myself. I have been afraid my whole life. But now, now I feel strong.

Lauren

The way I see things has felt like a burden throughout my life. I often seem to take things to places that make others feel uncomfortable or annoyed. I can't seem to go with the flow the way others do. I can't seem to let go of the injustice of the situation. It can sound very noble on paper but in reality, it is alienating and can be unbearably agonising, like I have a whole museum of pain that no one cares enough to look at. It is destabilising. *What I'm really trying to say is* the way I see things is often from a state of hypervigilance. It took me a long time to understand this. I couldn't understand why I was this way. It felt like a fatal flaw, and I still think it is quite often, but I try to fight this perspective. I wonder if the way I see things would be different if I knew what was being done to me then was wrong. If I had told someone. Would the compounding trauma of my youth and adulthood have occurred? This is a dangerous thought path to go down, one that fills me with enormous feelings of grief and loss, the loss of a life I could have lived, of potential I never got the chance to explore. It keeps coming into my head, one scene in particular. It was in a cupboard under a child's bunk bed, filled with dress ups and toys, that my childhood was violently fractured, my development and vitality compromised. A scene of innocence and imagination and play imbued with violation. An activity of free and fearless childhood expression was associated with disempowerment, confusion, and shame. Maybe that explains why the paths I have been drawn to have felt so confusing. I am drawn to expression and creativity and I get a thrill from ideas and critical thought, but my pursuit of these things has always felt unsafe. I knew where I felt most alive, but I was robbed of the safety to claim it as my space, to own my own expression. I felt wrong and displaced. I knew where I wanted to be and what I cared about but could never seem to feel at ease there. Since I have understood these things the possibilities for my life feel enlarged. I still have these feelings but there is a context, and a scene of trauma that I can see they are derived from.

I see you | When you see me | I hear you

Khale

I see you curled in a tight little ball at the foot of the bed. I see you crying in your car for the fifth time today, parked on a side street where you hope no one will see you. I see you pulling your long sleeves on to hide all the bruises on your arms. I see you hiding under a blanket in the living room because you are so scared of the shouting in the next room. I see you hunched over and plucking hairs out one by one as though it will somehow help. I see you scurrying between classes, clutching that sketchbook full of morbid drawings close to your chest. I see you hiding in the walk-in freezer just to escape for a few minutes from the leers and comments of those teenage boys. I see you desperately trying to befriend those women at the bar as though they will somehow protect you from the men who want you to explain why women falsely believe there is more than one way to orgasm. I see you hunched at your desk writing furiously by the light of the bare bulb, spilling all your shame into a journal that you keep so well hidden. I see you reading that journal years later and having vivid flashbacks of dirty encounters which somehow your brain has repressed for a decade.

What I'm really trying to say is, why do you always look like such a victim. Why are you always crying, or hurting yourself, or writing something shameful or hiding. Why do I never see you standing strong and proud. Why do I never see you fighting. Why do I never see you happy.

She sees you strong. She sees you fight. She sees you happy almost every day. She knows you in a way you don't even know yourself. So, when you think of yourself, remember yourself, why are you always a victim. Always sad, always alone, always full of shame, fear and regret.

Why don't you see all the good things when you look in the mirror? Why don't you see your laughter, your joy, your strength, your growth. Why do you define yourself by all your darkest hours. Why can't you start writing your story from scratch, and this time it's none of the bad stuff. Only light and love and happiness. Why can't you begin again, and this time be someone different.

Julie

When you see me I'm hidden away

When you see me I really want to say

You can never get inside my head

My thoughts are racing

And my voices want me dead

I wish so much

That people could see

What's behind my mask

And see the real me

I come across so quiet and shy

But my insecurities never reach the sky

I always wonder, what people think

Do I really care

Is that the real me

Why can't they see

That I have a good heart

And don't take advantage

I talk to my parts

When you see me

I crumble and fall

My words are broken

And I stumble to my knees

Please take time

To see what I mean

I don't want to fail

And let people down

But who's really hurting

I look all around

I need to be true to myself

And always shed doubt

Doubt comes from within
I'll shy away and go within
I feel alone
On the inside and out
I shed the kilos
But still there is self-doubt
Body image is important to some
But it's not the be all and end all
In this crazy world of glum
Crazy on so many levels
Crazy in my head
Crazy all around
Now the world is changing
Is it really round
I'm not making sense
And I try to write it down
But my words are jumbled
Frantically writing on pages
With my thoughts all scattered
Why can't I say what I feel
I feel totally shattered
FUCK nothings helping
There's so much to say
Why can't they see me
Maybe I'll pray
Pray, down on my knees
I'm really begging please
Please let the world see
I can only be me

Donna

I hear you

I see you

I listen to myself

When you see me

I hear you inside my head, it's damaging.
    You berate me, tell me I am disgusting and no good

I hear you crying, calling out for help,
    convinced it will never come

I hear you giving up, I hear you fighting, screaming.
    I see you discarded

I hear you, gentle heartbeat, oozing madness

Writhing in mud

I hear you break thy bone

I hear you confusing me, I lose consciousness

I sense something is not right, I am unsure
    how to think it through

I hear you shine a light in my face, yell close at me, terrorize me

I see you in darkness

I see you when it rains

I see you hiding in trees

I hear you question me

I hear you say she has no idea

I hear you say she is nothing

I hear you choose to side with them

I hear you choose to give up

I hear you choose to never let them win

I hear you choose to violate

Long drawn curtain blinds

Relax into breath

Gently roll over into dough

Disappear into moonlight

The sound of trees. A howling wind

Branches crack necks

I hear a bellowing cry, sickness

I can't see you

Time is created to skirt around the edges

Am I cutting into truth?

Will I ever make sense of it?

Is it possible to re-experience the pain?

I used to drink whisky

I used to drink to sleep

I used to drown my sorrows

Now I name them

Like a sober lament

As though pressing forward is worthwhile

Because, because, because

As though carrying on is essential

If so, if so, if so

As though naming it gives release

So, they say, so they say, so they say

I hear you tell me to write these words

I see you give expression to the interior

I hear you tune in, then disconnect

It's automatic, a glitch

Stuck. A hammer banging against the wall in the wind.

Rage | I am angry

Khale

Rage is wrong. I am not allowed to feel rage, but I want to.
I am not allowed to be angry, yet I can feel it deep inside me.
I am not allowed to yell and scream, yet it is bubbling within me.
Rage is wrong. Rage is not for girls. Then why do I feel like
I could tear down buildings with my screams? I want to punch,
to shout, to throw, to destroy. I am so so angry, but I am still
trying to be a good girl. How can I be both?

Lauren

I'm enraged and I can feel it building. I feel betrayed by
what's being said. The shrinking gap between the topic
of conversation and my very worth as a person is beating
loudly and the fury builds. I have to let it out. I try to breathe.
I storm out. Another moment for people to frame a picture
of me as hysterical, *not quite right*.

Donna

Rage is a machine inside me

That fuels my being

It is a distant wall

I am yet to cross over

It is exhaustion

RAGE is the low belly fire

I get when I hear your stories and learn what they did to you

And how you were forced to be complicit

RAGE stirs within me and cries to be released.

Julie

Rage what does that mean

Rage is so very foreign to me

Rage is something I wish I had

Rage was taught it's so very bad

Rage scares me

What will I become

If I let my defences down

Rage is what I fear

Rage can conquer my demons

Rage god help me

I'm full of fear

Nikki

I was taught that anger was bad, not for me.
    But fuck, that makes me livid.

I may be gentle, flighty, kind — but inside the simmering
rage monster lurks. After years of repressing it, I'm learning
to befriend my little monster — and ride it into the fiery battle
— now we fight together, me and my rage monster.

Julie

I am angry

Am I

So much abuse

Over so many years

No wonder my heart is full of tears

Am I angry

People try to explain

I don't understand

Anger is such a name

I am angry

I want to shout

I want to punch at their heads

And let my rage come out

I am angry

But only on the inside

Khale

I am angry at every disgusting man that sought to make
me feel small or embarrassed or intimidated. I talked with
a friend about all the times when we were young when men
would rub up against us on the bus or touch themselves or flash
us. Fuck those guys! What disgusting wastes of human beings!
Fuck those perverts, I want to kick every one of them in the nuts.
They are small, pathetic, disgusting losers.
I want to punch them all.

Lauren

I am angry that you won't fucking hear me. I can spell it
out clear as day and you still don't hear me. You discard
my pain and avoid responsibility. I resent you. For being well,
for not having demons, for being connected. I wish it was seen
as worthy of your time to see me, in all my disparate parts.
It's so easy for people to see you.

Dove

I'm angry I survived, that I exist, that I have to live with
what was done to me. I am angry there is no support for SRA,
I can't even find somewhere to live while they swan around
living it up with their money, cars, houses and reputations.

I'm angry I was born. I'm angry because it is preferable
to feeling the debilitating pain that lies underneath.

Donna

I am angry that I believed them

I am angry they took my power

I am angry I gave them power

I am angry they hurt my brain and stopped me from thinking

I am angry I hated me and not them

I am angry

I am angry

I am angry

I am angry

I am angry

I am angry that I am not angry.... that I cannot feel angry

But I'm angry that they say "she is angry"
    because they are seeing something I can't fully feel yet.

Being there for others | In its place On the way

Lauren

It's important to me to be there for others; to show up, to listen, to empathise. I have often invested too much in other people's pain, as though if I don't fully immerse myself in the depth of it I am at some level ignoring it, failing to bear witness to it. It's a rapid way to drain emotional resources. But I'm getting better at it. I think this is down to a few different factors, an important one being I'm valuing my own needs more, where I have routinely devalued them, as though sacrificing my needs is a requirement for caring. I've also developed more of a muscle for compassion over empathy, of staying closer to the boundaries of my own reality while still acknowledging the pain of others and showing care. I no longer think of myself as a horrible uncaring person for not showing up for everyone and everything. I can see this rationally makes sense. You can't identify problems clearly, and therefore provide the most appropriate support or assistance, if you activate your own survival brain. I know this from my own experience. The best help I receive when I'm in that place is the help conceived by people using their thinking brain, and generously supporting me in practical ways that help me move through it and regain my sense of safety. A home cooked meal. A change of scenery, taking me to the beach. Reminding me what is going on, kindly and patiently. Helping me see beyond the moment. It takes time to know what someone in crisis needs. It requires a relationship and a sense of trust. *What I'm really trying to say is* as a society we forget or are disincentivised from taking that time. We start to panic if someone honestly states how they feel that they are struggling. We find excuses not to engage, hiding behind rarely interrogated norms like *professional boundaries* or *social expectations*, finding comfort in the idea that it's someone else's job. I don't live my life in that world, and I think that's the only way out of it. It's something that survivors of all kinds of traumatic experience can lead the way on and do lead the way on. To be kind, truly kind, is radical *(thank you Jen Cloher)*. To be truly kind is to invest in others as a life practice, not a momentary kind word. That's why it is radical. I truly believe that, and I feel lucky to be surrounded by a tribe of people who practice it.

Julie

Being there for others

Seems an endless task

Wants, needs and more

Always running on empty

There are days in my life

I am so glad I have my wife

Keeping me focused

And talking out loud

I really don't want my head in the clouds

Always someone who needs a little more

More than I can give

But always needing the gig

I reach out my hand

And hope they understand

I am always there

In a capacity to bear

Such negativity comes from the outside

I'm lifting them up

And trying not to drown

Trying to be positive

For everyone else

I leave my own thoughts

On the top shelf

Life has thrown me

So many curveballs

From a very early age

I tried to reason

Only to fall down

And grapple with my thoughts

Every day I battle the voices

Never letting the outside in

I battle alone

Some people ask questions

And then suck them back up

Not really realising

I'm down on my luck

Why ask

When they don't really want to know

Know the truth

Of what happens in my head

I wish my face

Could really be read

Being there for others

Is something I do

It sometimes makes me feel

That they're human to

I sometimes let people in

Then shut myself down

I don't want the world to know

What's really happening

Out on my own

I'm feeling so sad

Deep within my heart

I don't let myself feel

The pain I felt from the start

I want to talk

And let my own feelings out

But I get shut down

And then I go inward

Alone with my thoughts

Talking in my head

And answering those voices

That I wish were dead

I'll always be someone that puts others first

Making sure of their well-being

And never letting them get hurt

Donna

In its place I fill the void

In its place I slumber

In its place I wrestle darkness

In its place, I swim lagoons of death

In its place I shake and rumble

In its place I beat drums

Burn fire

In its place I watch, mouth open

In its place I hide mouse quiet

In its place I bury under covers

In its place I dream foggy nightmares

Rose bush thorns

In its place someone shuffles

Do they feel guilt?

In its place I become all they should be

I become fault lines

I become dirt, filth

I become silence

I become evil

In its place is meant to be worship

In its place is wholeness

In its place is softness

In its place is stroked tears

In its place is what should have been

I become tender

I become gentle light

I become helper

In its place I let go of madness

In its place I break fear

In its place I step on darkness

In its place I smash vitriol

In its place I twist lies, throw truth

In its place I punch, hook your sickness

In its place I peek out frightened

In its place I stand master high

In its place I step in for you

In its place I hold out my hand

In its place I lift you all up

In its place I wave to the sky

In its place I cartwheel

In its place I fling my body

In its place I cough up wrongdoing

In its place I throw up your blood

In its place I nurse thy children

In its place I sing sweet songs

In its place I care for you

In its place I am tender

In its place I learn self-care

In its place I practice walking

In its place I beat my head

In its place I scream rage

In its place I break down

In its place I surrender

In its place I collapse

In its place I shudder

In its place I transform

In its place I am reborn.

Claire

On the way to the bathroom I feel the walls make my-self in the morning feel the walls in the hall through cold walls around me make a house on the way to a windy sitting at the computer of a day of unravelling the dreams that drag me down like someone took the plug out on my way to make myself a tea into the garden on my way to deciding I am not a victim it feels like punitive parenting and punishment but it is what I decide it is on my way to self-made get out of being caught in the fishing net of my fathermotherchurch and cruel cement drive way down the side of the house and screaming constriction on my way out of hell don't tell me anything anything at all leave me the fuck alone on the page where I am on the way to the bottom of the page and then another page turning the pages rereading the pages torn and turned toasted in the warmth of on my way to making a self every step in front of step forms a self to sacrifice to on my way to walking is hard lying on the ground on the way to the next class the next teaching on the way to the bathroom on the way to making on the way to becoming and unmending on the way to sitting and writing on the way to feel the peace of not trying on the way to all will be alright it can be alright on the way back on the way forward to what to the cliff edge no more ways there are no more aways no more waying no more weighing there is no more on the way there is just staying to know what staying is in to more on the way no more on the way just staying no more out of self no more getting somewhere no more being somewhere no more in the car driving between places between times between spaces on the way staying I am on the way staying hold both in the cup of my hands there will always be leakingthroughfingers on the way back on the way forward no more on the way way the on weigh the way way the way on the way I look out the window on the way I feel the warmth of the sun on the way the way there is no way there are ways and whys and hows and light wells and stairs and windows and cars and driving and sitting while fingers move on the keyboard on the way to finishing a timed exercise on the way to reason on the way to forgiving there is no on the way to forgiving there is just forgiving in degrees like pouring water into a cup there is a little bit then there is more there is no on the way on the way on the way the way is a path is it cliché yellow is it winding it is a way through the thickets it is a path down to the beach it is between two places two insides to places two owned spaces to labelled spaces the way has no label.

I pretend | I was tricked | Don't disturb

Lauren

I am very good at pretending, but it can be hard to tell if I'm pretending or just think I'm pretending and then I lose track of the baseline. Is there a baseline? If everyone is pretending all the time why do I feel so alone in so many situations? I pretended to be too smart for the high school social groups. I was the thinking, serious kid, the one with religious parents. I pretended I found it all easy, that it came naturally, that I didn't have to run myself into the ground to get an A+ or face the depths of my self-loathing. I pretended I just wasn't sporty, that I was clumsy, uncoordinated, when really I just didn't *get* my body. I couldn't make it move like the netball girls. I couldn't get past the fear and shame to focus on a game. Learning to run was a revelation, because I liked it and no one could watch me. I pretended to be really interested in getting fit and healthy. As I became thinner and thinner I told myself I was in control. If I felt I was losing control, the answer was more rules. Oh, the safety of rules. I pretended I was rebellious, drinking and smoking with the cool kids, but really I didn't get it. I pretended to have lofty aspirations and confidence, but I often thought I would die young. I pretended to be an adult, to be enjoying university. I pretended to be a free, fun-loving, drinking, funny cool girl. I pretended to like casual sex, to enjoy attention from men who were gross. I pretended to trust them. I pretended I was empowered when really I was buried. I pretended to be a professional, a grown-up. I worked hard, set parameters for myself, put rules in place. I pretended to loathe the idea of a long-term relationship, when I think deep down I felt I would never find someone willing to be with me. I couldn't see myself, how could someone else see me? My relationship with my partner has been a process of shedding. He was always interested in the stuff I wasn't pretending about. Over many years

I have learnt to feel safe. Our relationship has become a house I can move in, I can feel unformed in, I can emerge in. I don't have to pretend. It is an anchor. It is wonderful. It scares me. I work hard to convince myself it isn't right, that I'm unworthy, that it will self-destruct, that I must be pretending, but this is less and less as time goes on. I pretend to have lofty aspirations. I do. But I also have tiny ones. To live in the private universe we have created, to feel joy and be safe. That's all.

Nikki

I have spent a lifetime pretending. Pretending to be ok,
pretending I'm not hurt, pretending I'm happy.
I'm kind of done with pretending.

What I really want to say is I don't think I've ever been dishonest,
but I have lied — lied to protect my abuser from retribution,
lied to protect others from my own feelings and experience.
Lied to myself.

I've pushed down the feelings, the experiences trying to make
sure everyone else is ok — not to share my grief, and sorrow
and madness unless I am sure they can understand and take
it without taking it on as their own.

I've used imaginary make believe as an escape all my life.
Even now if I need to soothe myself I put on an audiobook
and pretend I'm safe — being read a bedtime story.
That feels real in a way that real life doesn't. I need it.
I need it like the brown cracked earth needs rain —
needs it to soften, recharge, renew. I need that soothing —
and I'm done pretending I don't.

What I really want to say is I am afraid, and tired. So very tired.

I have made a decision to stop pretending to be okay when
I'm not. To say "actually, I haven't slept, and I am stressed,"
instead of, "I'm great thanks. But how are you?" Pretending
to be okay, and deflecting concerns — I wonder if I can put
these as core skills on my resume? They feel more appropriate
than *proficient with the Microsoft suite.*

What I really want to say is I think the part that pretended
to be ok might have fallen asleep during lockdown.
A new part — or maybe the same? It's hard to know.
But they have started to respond with honesty
— sometimes brutal. But the old guilt and shame
that I used to feel didn't come.

And I didn't pretend.

Claire

I pretend I am a containable person, have a stable self, a coherent self, just listen to her friend, watch the fountain, the solar fountain I bought in salvaged bowl on salvaged green and repainted white, being both, pretend wrought iron table in backyard, sit on ground that might help, on the pretend ground being a pretend person, take her around my garden, my pretend sensory garden, smell the herbs I have planted to smell every morning when I have a pretend cup of tea, in the morning, pretend it does not help, it does help, I pretend I am a teacher, I pretend I am a friend, I pretend I am containable, I pretend I have a stable self, it helps to pretend, I pretend I do not recognize my own self, the things around me, what is that, it is when I am not in this time, I am in another time, a time robbed of being, I pretend because what else is there to do, it's good to pretend, to perform a self, to make remake make again a fluid and fatally flawed bowl of water, a shattering bowl of water that will take the shape of what I place it in, pretend I am in the shape of friend and teacher, I smell the herbs too, pretend it works before it takes some effect, pretend I make a life to live in to inhabit, I pretend I do not recognize myself, I do recognize myself, this self of no escape from trauma, I pretend I want to be an individual not this leaky bag of symptoms that can be prescribed to me by others who have experimented on knowing me, I pretend I don't care that I am pathologized, I pretend I do not care about who owns this information, I pretend I don't care I am limited to this, I pretend I don't care that doctors trauma therapists know more about compassion to me, I pretend I am an individual when I am a symptom, I pretend that is not true, I pretend this is news to me, I pretend it is inescapable, I pretend it is not too much reality, too reductionist, I pretend I am ok with this, I pretend there is not a way out of this bag. I pretend there is no bag, I pretend I am not lost so I can pretend I am finding, I pretend there is no time on the clock I pretend this does not matter, I pretend it is escapable, I pretend that not remembering works, I pretend I am more than this, I pretend I am not reduced to this is what a human with my life experience is, I pretend there are no commonalities, I pretend it is of my making, I pretend I am not made I make, I need to keep pretending that is what creating is pretending I am till I am. I am pretending

Khale

I was tricked into feeling safe. It is so easy to trick someone so small. We are so trusting. All we know is love and comfort and only the most occasional little hurts. My small life had been uneventful. I was at my favourite place in the whole world. The cabin by the beach where we went on holiday every year. All my days filled with sand and sea and playing with all my cousins whose families filled up all the other cabins. An annual festival where the entire tiny village was filled just with family. Just with people who loved me. That's what I believed with my whole tiny heart. I was tricked.

It's taken me years to remember all the pieces I know now. Every small detail is revealed to me in horrifying flashbacks. I remember, but not enough. Not enough to prove anything.

Every night, after the kids have all played until they are exhausted and been tucked into bed, the adults all gather into one cabin to play cards. I'm small, maybe four, but it's OK, the adults are not far away. I fall asleep easily because I am in a safe place. I was tricked into feeling safe here.

I wake up in the dark. I know I'm not supposed to be awake. I can see the wooden panels on the walls, the tacky ceiling. I can hear the clanging of the metal bed frame. I am not supposed to be awake in the dark. But I am, suddenly, and my body is flooded with bad feelings. I can barely breathe. He is on top of me and he is so heavy. I don't know what is happening. I am hurting, hurting in a place I have never felt anything before. My eyes are wide open. I want to make noise. I guess I do, because then those flannelette sheets with the pink and green stripes are on my face, in my mouth. I can barely breathe. He is so heavy. I hurt. I think I am going to die. Children are not supposed to hurt, to die. I don't understand who is doing this. I can see his moustache but I can't understand his face. I hurt, I hurt.

Suddenly I am gone, the room is gone, the pain is gone, I am no longer there. I escape. Whatever happened gets buried so deep in my tiny brain that I will not start to remember it again until I am 25.

It has come back to me in small pieces, in horrible flashbacks, how I was tricked. But never enough to know the full story.

Donna

I was tricked into silent submission, to believe foul mouths,
     leery eyes. I was tricked to reject body, be body,
     give body, despise body, use body.

I was tricked into saying I love you.

I want you.

I need you.

I deserve it.

I was tricked into believing I was ugly, worthless, filthy,
     a good for nothing, stupid slut.

I was tricked into lying for you,
     saying everything was good, okay.

I was tricked into following you.

I was tricked into blank thoughts.

What I really want to say is, what I really want to say is,
     what I really want to say is.

I was tricked into riot thinking.

Trauma short tripped my brain.

Razor sharp prods in my skin send currents to the networks
     of my mind.

I was tricked into acting older, mature, beyond my years
     when I was just a baby.

I was tricked into being some wild child, rebel, bad ass, evil.

I was tricked into wearing tiny shorts.

I was tricked into not eating, into starving my body so thin.

I was tricked into not feeling, keeping so busy,
     trauma runs through my veins.

Adrenalin rush.

Move quickly, onto the next thing, follow the light, slow down,
     run again to the next point.

I was tricked into death, into wanting vampires
  to come into my bed at night.

I was tricked into being bad, so it is the only time I feel alive.

I was tricked — betrayed — so I learnt to betray others.

I was tricked into separation, so connecting with others feels
overwhelming and foreign and I prefer to be alone.

I was tricked to build fantasy worlds in my head
  Rich, intoxicating, wild adventures, lost for days.

I was tricked to think you were smarter, funnier, kinder,
more considerate, more worthy, more loving, more beautiful,
wittier than I could ever be. I was tricked to keep it all buried
inside, so when bad dreams plagued me, I would go down for
days and backstage, the lights would go out, the theatre would
be empty, and I was the only one left inside until I exited
the back door, having forgot my lines, never to go back,
to perform the endless monologue.

I was tricked into thinking it was going to be alright,
but it is going to be alright, it always is alright, eventually.
Because life distracts, books, television, the internet,
more rabbit holes, until emptiness is felt again. That feeling
of I am back here again, how did I get back here again?
I try to remember what my therapist says — draw, write,
hold myself and I choose to consider the options, yet I have
forgotten how to act.

Julie

Don't disturb while my mind is so active

Don't disturb or I'm afraid I will cark it

When my mind is full

My body is always pulled

Pulled in directions, I have no time or space

Deep in my thoughts

Only time could erase

Don't disturb was what echoed all around

Don't disturb while I'm lying on the ground

I wish somebody did disturb

Every time I was there

I go deep inside myself

Knowing it's not fair

I won't let you in

Don't disturb

I choose to ignore

Don't disturb

The man in the shed

He'll only get angry

And go off his head

The phone rang one day

I wasn't even home

The call was for me

But little did I know

She jumped off the rocks

And came down with a thud

It was all my fault

I chose to run

Runaway and hide under a bridge

I hit the bottle

Now my body wasn't rigid

Only my thoughts and voices

Playing havoc with my digits

Don't disturb, as I lay alone

Scared and frightened

I won't make a noise or groan

Days went by and the bridge was my friend

And another bottle

I'm at my wits end

The time would come

When I returned home

Only to be yelled at

And beaten, now I'll groan

Don't disturb, was what was on my door

I don't want anyone to see I was so forlorn

Don't disturb I put barriers up

Don't disturb, but I'll never give up

Dove

Don't disturb the balance, the order, the secrecy. Don't disturb the dark, hidden secrets, open *Pandora's box*, expose the world to the evil that has been hidden for so long.

Don't disturb the ritual or else there will be severe punishment, death, chains and shackles. Blood, so much blood, it will be your fault.

Don't disturb the customer by crying, begging them to stop, don't disturb the fantasy little slut.

Don't disturb the video by crying or expressing pain, consequences are severe. Unless we want you to scream, then scream loud, don't disturb our enjoyment.

Don't disturb the assessment, failure means you must be punished, others punished, the babies punished, death, blood, torture, a fight, you'll have to do it again.

Don't disturb the family or coven, don't try to speak out, you are programmed to hurt yourself if you do, then we will hurt you and others worse.

Don't disturb their plans by daring to get pregnant and don't fight the abortion, it is your fault.

Don't disturb the memories, you don't know how much evil is hidden there. The dam breaks, a crushing avalanche buries me and all those who hear it.

Don't disturb others' safe, happy bubbles, blissful denial with your ugly horror. That cannot possibly happen in Melbourne, Australia, anywhere.

Don't disturb the belief that evil cannot walk among us unnoticed. It must be obvious, ugly, black, it cannot hide in plain sight.

Don't disturb the enjoyment of the predators, men who want to continue to use and abuse you, by breaking programming and saying no. Society needs used shells like you for men to play with so their sadism is hidden away from the rest of society.

Preferred ways of being
Prescribed ways of being

Donna

1 cup of kind, heart giving; softly knead

1 pinch of gentle, clever icing; shaken

1 tbsp of sincere goodness; meld into

½ cup laughing magic; sliced

Turn oven on

Wash hands for 20 seconds

Bake until burnt.

Nikki

Feel like I constantly strive for moment of calm, of serenity,
of stillness. I prefer a place where I can enforce my boundaries
physically — the walls of my house, my bedroom door.
In some ways I've discovered I like working from home —
no one can appear behind me; I can reject a call.

I prefer the company of one or two other people,
with one-on-one being my favourite. It limits the emotions
I can take on.

I prefer.

What I really want to say is, I prefer.

Khale

My preferred way of being would be to be an entity.
A ball of energy. A soul. I can communicate, I can feel,
I can listen, I can hold space. But none of the baggage
that comes with this body. No breasts, no hips, no bum,
nothing that people want to touch. Sometimes I dream
of being genderless — of people not automatically perceiving
me as *woman*. But then, that also makes me a target. Other.
"Fucking fag." Why can't I just exist? Why does a body have
to be something to want or hate or fight? Why can't I just be?
I want to be noticed but also, I am terrified of being perceived.

Lauren

It's ok to talk passionately but not too passionately.
Don't overdo it. Remember you know nothing.
You are nothing. You need to prove yourself but don't
over-prove. You'll overwhelm people. Everyone is doing
their best. You can have expectations but make sure they
are realistic. That's not how the world works. That's not
how people are. Boys need extra help to talk about their
emotions and to clean the house. Make sure you don't assert
yourself too much, keep your head down, pick your battles.
Don't be naive. Remember at the end of the day most people
only care about themselves.

Nikki

Be thinner, be smarter, be softer, be stronger

Be funny, be desirable, be *not like the other girls*, be cool,
    be hot, be up in the sky and be down to earth

Be right, be left, but at the same time

Be ok, be open, but keep your thoughts to yourself

Be thinner, but let me take your picture

Be more, be everything. You are inadequate
    and have been found wanting

Be better, newer, younger, more mature.
    Be energetic, never tired, never boring

Be.

Khale

I made a decision to listen to doctors, mostly because
my girlfriend was so terrified of what I had become.
Take your meds, all of them. Go to therapy, go often.
See the dietitian. Eat everything, *eat, eat, eat*.
Eat until you can stand. Eat until your brain recovers.
Eat until you can walk through the cold aisle
at the supermarket without freezing to death.
Take your meds. Talk about it. Speak your secrets out loud.
Doesn't that feel better? No! I hate it. I am so ashamed.
Wouldn't it have been better if I had just faded away to nothing?
Please stop making me talk about it. I am so ashamed.

Donna

Nice, calm, soft, gentle

Full of *joie de vivre*

Hop, skip, jump

Light and fluffy

Good cook

Clean

Organised

Into sports

Hiking

Long walks on the beach

Gluten free

Free range

Hetero-normative

Inclusive

Radically full of love

Radical love

Innovative and dynamic

Flexible

Go with the flow

Supportive

Adaptive

Critical thinker

Smart enough to beat the robots

Thoughtful.

The Unknown | The Atmosphere

Khale

I think there is a world that other people experience that is so separate from me. I learn about it from my wife. She meets people and assumes the best of them. In her experience, most people are good. Most people don't hate you or want to hurt you. She moves about the world and feels relatively safe. She does not spend hours of every day obsessing or spiralling into an anxious pit.

I don't know how to get to this other world. I was born into something different. Where I live, you can't just trust people. You don't feel safe. You can't close your eyes. Your mind can't rest. My world is so different.

It seems so random and unfair that some of us live in a world where bad things happen, over and over again, and some of us just get to live — happily, peacefully, never worrying about where the next bad thing is coming from.

Maybe I was someone terrible in a past life and my wife was a saint.

Lauren

I don't like not knowing. It is uncomfortable. If I misplace something or a weird thing happens that defies logic, it bothers me and niggles at me. Probably why I'm obsessed with the way things work, why I studied philosophy. But then this opened the unknown, and now I know the more I know the more I don't know, the less I trust people who claim to know. What is it to know? Can we really separate ourselves from our knowing? What on earth am I trying to say? I often think about this when I receive reactions of scepticism or surprise at how intimately I understand my mental illness, as though the illness should stop me knowing, or that for some reason knowing means it should no longer have a hold on me. To know is not to be, but it helps make sense of the being. I will not give up my space and my right to know the things that influence my being. I will not accept the notion that my ability to know is compromised by my being.

Nikki

My immediate response was the un-NOOOOOOOOOO-wn.

The unknown terrifies me — I have no way of knowing what will happen, or how I'll react. Just thinking about it — I can feel my heart race, my shoulders hunch, the sweats start, and the barriers come up. I am a person who religiously re-watches the same shows and re-reads the same books — because I know what will happen. I have control and that's comforting.

But I also know that the unknown, while scary, could hold beautiful things. I met my partner through taking a chance on an unknown university course.

Each of those books and shows had a first time, a first chance. Maybe I need to release some control and jump into the chasm of unknown — limbs outstretched and trust that these opportunities might be worth it.

Donna

The unknown was a terrifying concept, it still is.

It used to be worse. I once needed to have a sense of control
and certainty over everything. I have done so many wild
things, escaping into the unknown, yet clamped down
on my life in so many other ways. It is hard to know if I live
in the unknown or run away from it. The thing I hate about
the unknown is that it is unknown, yet it drives me, us, it,
like our unconscious. The unknown is *known*, a *gnome*,
buried in a garden, waiting to be dug up, a treasure box
of repressed memories that defies censorship. The unknown
is *known*, it is *grown*, inside my head, until it stares out in front
of me.

Nikki

The atmosphere has shifted and is in flux. The mist swirls, descending, cascading, lifting, shifting with the shifts in emotions and desire — so deeply held they aren't ever articulated outside therapy.

The mist shifts.

'I don't ever want children' — I bluster, throw out the statement, and mean it. I love children, but I don't want, need my own. I would be happy being an aunt, a friend — someone safe, a port in the storm. I want to be for a child, what I wish I had had when I was small. Someone to be there — to notice. To not be so wrapped up in all the affairs and *to dos*, to notice when they were sad, scared, worried. To be there and teach them, *it's ok not to get it right*, perfect isn't desirable — learning and reflection are.

What I really want to say is this is something I've wanted for as long as I can remember. It's deep and visceral — I want to nurture. But I can't even keep my fucking house plants alive. Like — it's a cactus, how is it dying?? Although maybe the problem is that they thrive on neglect — and that's the opposite of how I'm inclined.

The mist shifts — I'm terrified of the longing to nurture. What if I become overbearing, too involved, too much? What if I don't?

It's partly why I've always said I don't necessarily want my own children — I don't want to fuck them up. If I am truly honest, I sometimes increasingly agree with my demonic uterus — I would love to have my own. But I am terrified I'd get it wrong. I'm so afraid that I'd be too much — and the worst fear — the deepest darkest, most turbulent part of the mist and pressure — is that I would become an abuser. It goes against everything I am, and I know that — but it still scares me.

I'd want to protect — but I'm aware that maybe I couldn't protect them from the behaviour I was modelled, the inadvertent lessons I was taught — the same ones I learnt at my grandmother's knee, and my grandfather's hands.

I say goodbye to | The last eight weeks

Khale

I say goodbye to feeling weak. I say goodbye to the body that couldn't run, got too out of breath, couldn't do a push-up. I say goodbye to always feeling afraid. I say goodbye to hiding inside for months because the world is a terrible place. I say goodbye to staying up all night because I'm afraid to fall asleep.

I say hello to my new body. The body that can run five kilometres easily, that can do real push-ups, that can punch and make an impact. I say hello to these legs that feel so firm when I squeeze them. I say hello to arms that are starting to look like something other than the wobbly limbs I always saw on my grandma.

This is a body I can feel good in. This is a body I can be grateful for. This is a body that is so capable, so strong, and finally, I feel worthy. With this body, I look forward to a weekend of working in the garden because I know I can dig for hours and sweat and puff yet keep going.

With this body, setting out for a run feels good, feels light, because I know I can make it. With this body, I can lift weights, I can help people move house, I can flip the mattress.

My body has transformed. I don't hate it anymore. I hated it for so long, all my life, because I felt so betrayed by it, like it always invited hurt.

I am sorry I treated you so badly. I am ready to be kind to my body. My body serves me. My body can move, can fight, can do so many things. I am so thankful that this body has managed to survive so long, despite everything.

Thank you, finally, to whatever those good good brain chemicals are. My moods have become so incredibly different. Anyone meeting me for the first time would think I was a naturally happy person, and that feels *so weird* to me. I've been depressed my whole life.

I feel like, for the first time, my brain and I are fighting on the same side. I laugh. I smile. I take joy. I am a strange new person who may even live a long life after all.

Thank you to my body. Thank you to my brain. Thank you to this journey which has brought me so much healing. Thank you to these wonderful people who have been so vulnerable, so kind. Thank you for holding space for me. Thank you for listening without judgement. Thank you for making me feel like I could be worthwhile. Thank you for cradling me so gently as I built myself up. Thank you.

Lauren

I say goodbye to the cynicism. The bad behaviour, the lack of kindness, camaraderie, community. I say goodbye to toxic leaders and self-labelled progressives who won't look at themselves honestly. I say goodbye to my preconceived notions about what this would or could be, what it meant for me, what it says about how I am. I say goodbye to people who won't back up their professed values with action. It fucking infuriates me. The cynicism sickens me. So, I'm using my power to let it go. I will not associate myself with it. As the crises of white imperialism, patriarchy and capitalism come to a head, to points so large and dire, I cannot be fucked caring about the conventional path anymore. Given what is at stake, why would I keep participating in this toxic machine that also makes me suffer? So, I say hello to the possibilities of another way. I say hello to community, to radical self-love. I say hello to art and ideas and thinking beyond the scaffolds of power and ideology. I say hello to joy and simplicity, to building a home in a tiny piece of the world, to growing my own food. To helping and holding the friends who see me, and who I see. To having boundaries with those who refuse to see. I say hello to finding my own way and my own voice, to throwing out the legitimacy of the old that has created this mess. I no longer feel destroyed by being labelled naive, which almost always comes from someone unwilling to have an honest conversation, to get to the heart of the matter. I want to live a life of getting to the heart of the matter, to finding the most human responses to the problems we are facing. I want to claim a voice for my unique experience while advocating for the dismantling of the systems of oppression that enabled it. Fuck it, I may as well make something of this. I often feel this way when I've hit rock bottom, that I may as well salvage something from the mess of my life. In itself it is a drive, a force that allows me to pick myself up again and find a way forward.

Julie

I say goodbye to a life I had known

I say goodbye to the people I once loved

It's time to go

And in a way I'm so thankful

Thankful, may not be the right word

But to a life that is ending

I spent all of my young years

In a country I loved

But to say goodbye comes with so many emotions

I'm leaving this place

And going far across the ocean

My life as a child was carefree and playful

Thinking this time would never end

I found myself

At my wits end

How can someone's life change so much

It only happened when my life just thrust

I was only eleven

When my world turned upside down

Who could have imagined

I'd spend the next two years on the ground

Everyday after school

I was tortured and raped

Each taking a turn

I hated going through the gate

After two long years

I was told with glee

We would be moving

Far across the sea

I would say goodbye

To the friend I had known

But I was filled with emotion

Of leaving and no more abuse

It couldn't come sooner

What would they do

Please don't find someone else to abuse

Finally, the time came

And we were packed and ready to go

If only I knew what my future would hold

I hated the new country

Kids were so cruel

Always being bullied

I felt like a tool

I finally made some friends

And things were OK

Until it happened again

Down the beach one day

How could this happen again

I asked all my voices

They said with delight

Always keep on your toes

You never know what happens in the night

I finally just sat

With the feelings within

I had a new life

But I longed to go back

And start once again

It's a tough old track

Finally, again we were moving back home

Away from the abuse

I had come to know

Gabrielle

In the last eight weeks one of my biggest fears was failure.
   I was terrified that I would fail the

compulsory editing subject for my Master's.

My life was about living in that fear and anxiety.

But surprise, surprise I passed the subject.

Now I am enrolled in the second and last compulsory
   editing subject for second semester.

Amazingly, studying is giving me a way to survive Covid.

Studying is giving me familiarity and resilience.

Something to live for in these trying times
   in this state of emergency.

What has the group given to you that you would like other survivors to know about?

Khale

This group has given me a space to be heard. To be safe. To let every dark, shameful secret that has haunted me out into the light and see that it doesn't always drive people away, shut them down. This group has allowed me to rinse my insides out, get some of that horrible grease off me. I feel accepted for the worst parts of myself. I always felt *if people really knew me, they would hate me*. But this group knows all the worst bits and yet they still smile at me, still say my name. This is a kind of acceptance that doesn't come easily. This is such incredible kindness. This is slow, sure healing. This is letting go.

Lauren

This group has given me a vocabulary to understand myself, and the safety to try to articulate it. Never had I met a group of women who could share my experiences of navigating the world with such honesty and grace. Women who have also felt like they are too much and not enough, like they look in at the world from some other vantage point. I feel more myself whenever I think about the women in this community. It is a refuge for the vulnerabilities that hold my being.

Julie

What the group has given to me

Is highs and lows

On a weekly basis

Sometimes I felt so alone

But now I have purpose

Boxing makes me feel strong

A group of strangers

Who are now so close

We bond in a way

Words sometimes aren't spoken

But we know in our hearts

The pain that we feel

We are never alone

I want others to know this

And open your hearts

Nikki

This group has given me comfort — a safe place to honestly
express all parts. A place to be holistic in my joy, shame,
and confusion.

We're all muddling through our own, and shared experiences
— buoyed up by each other.

 I want other women to be able to experience
this sense of connection and understanding.

To feel the love and safety this group provides.

I want them to feel safe to be vulnerable, safe to be strong,
safe to rage.

Donna

Inspiration. Heart. Power. Strength. Funny. Stories. Play. Comfort. Solidarity. Fear. Agency. Vulnerability. Protection. Love. Passion. Connectedness. Anger. Anger. Anger. Words. Language. Ideas. Motivation. Joy.

Epilogue

The *Left/Write//Hook* workshops continue to run each year and I am looking to expand the program on a national and international scale.

This will involve training both boxing and writing facilitators to work with groups. My aim is to create a trauma-informed boxing and arts-based space to hold the workshops and other creative arts programs for survivors.

The key research findings from the first round of the *Left / Write // Hook* program provide evidence that the combined acts of creative writing and boxing assist survivors of childhood sexual abuse and trauma in their recovery and wellbeing. The workshops created a space for survivors to disclose their abuse without judgement and to consider (re)storying their experiences through creative writing and the embodied activities practiced within boxing. For those who attended each week, the data showed that their assertiveness increased over time. The participants demonstrated improvements in PTSD symptoms and their overall well-being. General symptoms of depression, anxiety, and stress also improved across the program, along with the survivors' sense of personal agency and relationship with others.

The implications of this research project are particularly important in the current political climate. In the wake of the #MeToo campaign, the rape allegations against various global leaders and the viral online petitions calling for an overhaul of sexual consent education in schools, the number of women who are speaking out about their experiences with sexual assault and violence is rapidly rising. Research reveals one in three women are abused before the age of 18 (Fergusson & Mullen, 1999). There is an urgent need to place the conversations of childhood sexual abuse and its effects on survivors into contemporary discourse about gendered violence. My hope is that this book will do just that.

Grace Tame, recipient of the Australian of the Year award for 2021, noted upon receiving her award that while discussion of childhood sexual abuse is uncomfortable; nothing is more uncomfortable than the abuse itself. Tame also said that survivor stories help to "redirect this discomfort to where it belongs — at the feet of perpetrators" (Gredley, 2021).

These conversations are needed now more than ever, and they need to be led by those with lived experience. As this project is founded in Melbourne, Victoria, Australia, it is pertinent to note the findings generated by the Royal Commission into Victoria's Mental Health System. Their recommendations state that the delivery of accredited training and resources need to be led by people with lived experience of mental illness or psychological distress (State of Victoria, Royal Commission into Victoria's Mental Health System, 2021).

Left/Write//Hook has made important strides in supporting survivors of childhood sexual abuse to feel creatively empowered to share their lived experiences in a holistic program that addresses both mind and body. Yet, broader questions remain, and other new questions have arisen. As I continue to build this program, I am left to wonder:

- What are the best ways to engage in participatory, holistic, and collaborative research to increase agency and amplify the voices of childhood sexual abuse survivors?

- What is the effect of survivor-led programs on the survivor community? How does this change or impact the survivors' experience and sense of agency?

- How can programs be co-created and co-researched by, with and for survivors?

- How can Left/Write//Hook be scaled to reach national and international level?

You can read the published journal article of the research findings here:
www.internationaljournalofwellbeing.org/index.php/ijow/article/view/1505

The documentary is still in production and you can track its progress here:
www.leftwritehook.com/

If you are inspired by this project and want to get in touch, please contact Donna at
leftwritehook@gmail.com

References

Fergusson, D & Mullen, P (1999), Childhood Sexual Abuse: An Evidence Based Perspective, Thousand Oaks: Sage Publications.

Gredley, R. (2021). Abuse survivor is Australian of the year. The Canberra Times, 25 January 2021

Lyon, D., Owen, S., Osborne, M. S., Blake, K., & Andrades, B. (2020). Left / Write // Hook: A mixed method study of a writing and boxing workshop for survivors of childhood sexual abuse and trauma. International Journal of Wellbeing, 10(5), 64-82. **doi.org/10.5502/ijw.v10i5.1505**

State of Victoria, Royal Commission into Victoria's Mental Health System, 2021. Royal Commission into Victoria's Mental Health System Final Report. Summary Recommendations. [online] Melbourne: Royal Commission into Victoria's Mental Health System, Melbourne Victoria. Available at: **<finalreport.rcvmhs.vic.gov.au/download-report/>** [Accessed 7 March 2021]

Contributor Bios

Claire Gaskin

Claire Gaskin's, *a bud* was released by John Leonard Press in 2006, and was shortlisted in the John Bray SA Festival Awards for Literature in 2008. Her collection *Paperweight*, was published in 2013 by Hunter Publishers. Her collection, *Eurydice Speaks*, was published with Hunter Publishers in 2021. *Ismene's Survivable Resistance* is forthcoming in 2021 with Puncher & Wattmann.

Dove

Dove is a survivor of satanic ritual abuse. She has spent years working through repressed memories and learning to live with her abuse and its impacts. She loves animals and hopes to work with survivors in an animal therapy program in the future.

Gabrielle

Gabrielle has a PhD in creative writing and has written two books of poetry. She has been published in numerous journals and anthologies and has performed her poetry nationally and internationally.

Julie

Julie is a 53 year old woman with many qualities. She endured years of child sexual abuse and has schizophrenia, which develops into trauma induced psychosis. She believes that her mental health does not define the person she is today. She is in a loving relationship of 30 years. Julie is loving and caring and has a passion for singing and the arts.

Khale McHurst

Khale is a queer autobiographical comic artist working on the lands of the Wurundjeri people of the Kulin Nation. Her work explores mental illness, queer relationships, and growing up in a religious cult. She enjoys a boring life with their wife and fur family.

Lauren

Lauren is an arts worker, intersectional feminist, sometimes writer, and graduate student who is interested in what it means to live our ethics publicly. She is a survivor of childhood sexual abuse and cancer. She lives with her partner and fluffy cat on the unceded lands of the Wurundjeri and Bunurong peoples, where she enjoys growing things in her tiny garden.

Nikki

Nikki is a mess — but a really optimistic one. She is an unapologetically huge nerd, living buoyantly with mental illness and the lasting impacts of her childhood sexual abuse. She is committed to being kind in a world that is not always so. She lives and works on the unceded land of the Wurundjeri people of the Kulin Nation.

Donna Lyon — Editor

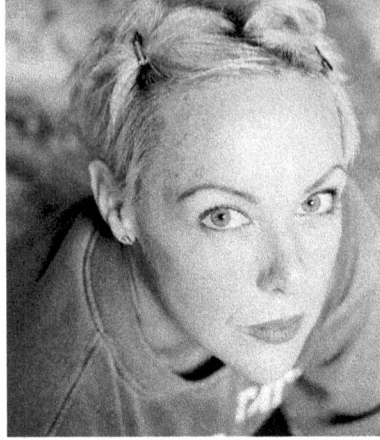

Donna grew up in Perth, Western Australia and is a survivor of ritual abuse. She has an impressive laundry list of symptoms, after years of battling with the psychological, physical, mental, and emotional effects from her trauma. It led her to a ten-year recovery journey where she found sobriety and God through spiritual and emotional healing. She is now a publicly declared child sexual abuse survivor, along with being a boxer, academic and multi-disciplinary producer. Her production background spans a variety of formats, including television, feature films, documentary and online content. Her film work has been screened nationally and internationally in film festivals in USA, Europe and Australia. Her recent feature film Disclosure (2020) had its world premiere at the 31st Palm Springs International Film Festival and at Adelaide Film Festival (2020). The film is released in the USA by Breaking Glass Pictures and in Australia and New Zealand by Bonsai Films. She is an alumnus of the University of Melbourne and now an academic there, working in the Film and Television department. She is a Senior Lecturer in the Master of Producing program and has just submitted her PhD. Donna is the founder of *Left / Write // Hook*, and her research interests now focus on the intersection of creative arts and sport on the mental health and wellbeing of survivors of child sexual abuse.

www.ingramcontent.com/pod-product-compliance
Lightning Source LLC
Chambersburg PA
CBHW070242200326
41518CB00010B/1650